I0786464

ASHLAND THEOLOGICAL SEMINARY

INTEGRATING GOD'S DIVINE WELLNESS PLAN TO IMPACT
CHRISTIAN WOMEN'S HOLISTIC LIFESTYLE IN CLEVELAND, OHIO

A DISSERTATION SUBMITTED TO
THE FACULTY OF ASHLAND THEOLOGICAL SEMINARY
IN CANDIDACY FOR THE DEGREE OF
DOCTOR OF MINISTRY

BY REVEREND FREDINA J. USHER-WEEMS

CLEVELAND, OHIO

MARCH 22, 2018

Gracednotes Ministries
405 Northridge St. NW
North Canton, Ohio 44720

Scriptures taken from the Holy Bible, New International Version®, NIV®.
Copyright © 1973, 1978, 1984, 2011 by Biblica, Inc.™
Used by permission of Zondervan.
All rights reserved worldwide. www.zondervan.com
The "NIV" and "New International Version" are trademarks registered in the United
States Patent and Trademark Office by Biblica, Inc.™

Copyright © 2018 by Fredina J. Usher-Weems
All rights reserved

Printed in the United States of America

ISBN-13:
978-1717394958

ISBN-10:
1717394957

To Byron Weems, my handsome husband and a man after God's own heart,
Estella Usher, my mother (who went home to be with the Lord in 2005),
Fred Usher, my father,
Pristella Usher and Rebecca Perry, my two sisters,
and Ivoe and LeAnder Nicholson, my adorable two nephews,
who have been my support system

I decided long ago, never to walk in anyone's shadows
If I fail, if I succeed
At least I'll live as I believe
No matter what they take from me
They can't take away my dignity
Because the greatest love of all
Is happening to me
I found the greatest love of all
Inside of me
The greatest love of all
Is easy to achieve
Learning to love yourself
It is the greatest love of all

(Lyrics by Whitney Houston: *The Greatest Love of All*)

ABSTRACT

The purpose of this project was to impact the healthcare of women within the Union-Miles community in Cleveland, Ohio by providing six weeks of holistic workshops that help participants integrate God's Divine Wellness Plan into their daily lives. Quantitative and qualitative pre-tests and post-tests were designed to assess knowledge related to the wellness lifestyles of the African American women participants.

The project revealed what the women learned and comprehended about God's health and fitness plan that balanced wellness components for the whole person. The project confirmed that the participants lacked the necessary Bible-based wellness tools to live in healthy ways.

CONTENTS

LIST OF TABLES

Table

ACKNOWLEDGEMENTS

This project was possible because of the contributions from many others. I am sincerely grateful and thankful to those mentioned below:

Giving honor to my Lord and Savior Jesus Christ who instilled within me the desire, compassion, and will to pursue my dream and vision to serve others within the community in the area of wellness.

To my loving, handsome husband, Byron Weems, who was my cheerleader, support person, and intercessor throughout the whole journey. Whether I felt energized, anxious, overwhelmed, or at peace, Byron always reminded me that my strength, will, and endurance rested in the Lord versus self.

To my father, Fred Usher, who unconditionally supported every idea, goal or dream I had since childhood.

To the memory of my mother, Estella Usher, who now resides with the Lord. She taught me work ethics and how to serve others with humility.

To my sister, Pristella Usher, who believed that in Christ I could do whatever I believed was possible.

To my sister, Rebecca Perry and her husband Herman Perry, who always supported me.

To my nephews, Ivoe and LeAnder Nicholson, who always spoke words of life into my dreams.

To my godmother, Margie Glass (went home to be with the lord in 2010) who walked close with God and encouraged me to walk close with God.

To my spiritual mentors, Janis Miles, Theron Kittnetes, and Renee Kittnetes, who always reminded me of what God's divine wellness plan was for me. They listened to my complaints, concerns and fears and reminded me to press on in Christ.

To my many prayer warriors, Emma Austin, Arlette Coulter, Quintene Frederick, Janis Hill, Philomena M. Johnson, Georgia Misener, Cheryl Nash, and Deonna Taylor, for being my Aaron and Hur throughout this dissertation season.

To my cheerleaders, Falana and Hannah Banks, Lisa Bostick, LaShorn K. Caldwell, Nelia Deskins, Calvin Grant, Connie Grant, Carlin Grant, Robin Houston, Theresa L. Johnson, Erica Marks, Vicki William Morrison, Bunda Russ, Andre Smith, Sherrion Smith, Hattie Weems, and John Weems (who went home to be with our Lord and Savior, 2016), who cheered me through the trials and tribulations encountered while pursuing my Doctor of Ministry program.

To my church family, The Church on the North Coast, for their words of encouragement, prayers, advertisement, and faith support.

To my editor, Dr. Matthew Bevere, I appreciated the many hours he spent reading and editing this project for me in love.

To my research support team members, Debra Lewis-Curlee (MS, LSW), Shuywanna Ford (MCMSW, BBS), Dr. Mladen Golubic, Kristin Kirkpatrick (RN), Bryan Pflaum (MFA), Edward R. Schmidthke (M.A. secondary Ela. Teacher), and Pastor Vontayne Smith, for spiritual and intellectual information they provided me.

To Dr. Donna Clemons, my field consultant, who enthusiastically volunteered for the role. She patiently, lovingly, and prayerfully offered constructive feedback.

To my advisor, Dr. JoAnn Shade, who lovingly checked on me throughout the process. I am grateful and thankful for her nurturance, support, and spiritual guidance through the writing and research of this project.

CHAPTER ONE

INTRODUCTION AND PROJECT OVERVIEW

You may write me down in history with your bitter, twisted lies. You may trod me in the very dirt but still, like dust, I'll rise. Does my sassiness upset you? Why are you beset with gloom? Cause I walk like I've got oil wells pumping in my living room. Just like moons and like suns, with the certainty of tides, just like hopes springing high, still I'll rise. Did you want to see me broken? Bowed head and lowered eyes? Shoulders falling down like teardrops, weakened by my soulful cries? Does my haughtiness offend you? Don't you take it awful hard cause I laugh like I've got gold mines diggin' in my own backyard. You may shoot me with your words. You may cut me with your eyes. You may kill me with your hatefulness, but still, like air, I'll rise. Does my sexiness upset you? Does it come as a surprise that I dance like I've got diamonds at the meeting of my thighs? Out of the huts of history's shame I rise up from a past that's rooted in pain I rise. I'm a black ocean, leaping and wide, welling and swelling I bear in the tide. Leaving behind nights of terror and fear I rise into a daybreak that's wondrously clear. I rise bringing the gifts that my ancestors gave. I am the dream and the hope of the slave. I rise. I rise. I rise. (Maya Angelou: *Still I Rise*)

Why were my professional qualifications not respected or accepted within white corporate America? Why must I continuously experience racial and gender inequality? Why should my empowerment, body image, and sexuality as a woman be defined through media stereotypes, from a history of slave entrapment, and from a male chauvinist's perspective? These are some of the questions I asked myself, and other African American women ask themselves, while on our journey of lifestyle identity. They ponder over their self-identity because they were exposed to negative lifestyle challenges such as unemployment, financial debt, sexual abuse, alcohol and drug addiction, homelessness, prison, spiritual depletion, low self-esteem and depression.

Because of their struggles with self-identity, African American women often struggle to take care of themselves. Yet I knew from my own experience, as well as from researchers such as Musgrave, Allen and Allen, that "the intersection of spirituality or religiosity and health for ethnic African American women can make a difference in their health experience, helping to eliminate health disparities and promoting positive health outcomes" (Musgrave, Allen and Allen 2002, 560).

In the development of this project, my God-given desire was to help African American women acknowledge their need for wellness assistance while benefiting from God's healthcare plan. Wellness unifies the whole person, uplifting the spirit, soul, and body. The Bible-based health and fitness plan that was the basis for this project was created to equip African American women spiritually, mentally, intellectually, and physically, because healthy, holistic living through God's word can result in increased inner peace for the African American women participants. Through this impact study, my hope was that their identity in Christ would be revealed, allowing them to build better families and assist their families in building better communities. Through this process, they would find ways to become better mothers, wives, and friends, finding self-value, self-worth, and self-esteem in knowing who they were in Christ.

Purpose Statement and Research Question

The purpose of this project was to impact the healthcare of women within the Union-Miles community in Cleveland, Ohio by providing six weeks of holistic workshops that help participants integrate God's Divine Wellness plan into their daily lives. The research question was: what impact will this six weeks of holistic workshops have on the healthcare of the women within the Union-Miles community in Cleveland Ohio?

Overview

Through this project, God inspired me to create a series of workshops for African American women called Diva's Lifestyle Identity Journey. The Diva's Lifestyle Identity Journey interactive workshops were designed to impact the healthcare of African American women through Bible-based sessions focused on education, motivation, and fashion. This project helped the women transition from their current identity struggles into women who were rooted within the stability of self-sufficiency in Christ. The six-week interactive workshops incorporated scripturally-based tools which energized the African American women both spiritually and physically.

The workshops were held once a week for three hours. The sessions were held on Saturday morning at a community center in Cleveland, and were designed to be interactive. They focused on:

Stress Release: helping the women release their frustration and give it to God.

Identity Crisis: helping the participants find their identity in God's love and answer the question, "who am I?"

Healthy Heart and Soul: helping participants effectively handle their emotional state through an honest, inward examination of their feelings.

Body Image and Fitness: helping participants overcome their negative images that link to diminished mental performance, low self-esteem, anxiety, sexual dysfunction, depression, and eating disorders.

Mouth Trap: helping participants choose their words in a manner that is fruitful and flows from their dreams and visions.

Dress for Success and Diva's Wrap Up: helping participants select dress attire that gave a visual image of who they appeared to be in Christ.

The weekly educational sessions helped the women know and accept their identity in Christ. The Diva's Proclamation used at the beginning of each session energized and reassured each woman of their identity in Christ, gave them a sense of self-awareness, and helped to clarify the purpose of their lives. The small group stress relaxation meditation exercises ushered the African American women into a peaceful, safe, and pleasant environment. The discussion period allowed the women to express their fears, concerns, prayer requests, and testimonies. The weekly homework assignments engaged and encouraged the women to use various wellness techniques throughout their daily interactions, both personal and professional.

Preliminary assessment tools were given to each participant, first as a pre-test, and then as a post-test. These written surveys were used to determine the participants' lifestyle practices and self-awareness in relation to God's word, physical activities, nutrition selections, stress management, self-identity, and soul-searching. The pre-test revealed their lifestyle choices before attending the workshops. The post-test results revealed how the workshops impacted their wellness lifestyle choices and awareness of God's word within their daily activities.

At the conclusion of the six weeks, the participants, their families, friends, and community members attended a free community fashion show called the Diva's Wrap Up session, designed to be their victory walk, in which they revealed their spiritual and physical transformation through their unique statements of fashion. The results were posted on a Facebook account called Inside/Out Diva's Lifestyle Identity Journey.

While not studied in this project, the program itself had a follow-up phase with a weekly evaluation that addressed the ongoing impact the participants experienced through the continuous application of the program. The follow-up gatherings were done online, through phone conversations, and text message. Comments were also made through an In/Out Diva's Lifestyle Identity Journey Facebook page. This format was convenient because the various careers of the participants made it difficult to gather together again. The Facebook site provided (and still provides) daily motivational tips, suggestions for ongoing health care education, prayer support, and accountability for growth provided through their feedback postings.

Foundations

Gems are hard stones, and these rough, hard stones need to be cut and all the flaws removed. Once cut, they are polished to add to their luster and increase their brilliance, to allow color to shine through, and to create "fire" or a rainbow-like sparkle. Your "fire" and your sparkle comes by such a process too. Your character flaws are removed as you work to eliminate what is not pleasing to God, all that hurts and harms others. And as you polish up your practical skills and gain greater emotional stability, you will indeed sparkle as you bless others and shine with God's brand of beauty. (George 2014,18)

In her book, *Beautiful in God's Eyes: For Young Women Looking Good From the Inside Out*, Elizabeth George presented a challenge to me: What would it look like for African American women in my community to capture their concept of shining "with God's brand of beauty" (George 2014, 18)? What would be the foundations for me personally? What biblical, theological, historical, and contemporary research could I include in my project that would allow me to design a Bible-based health plan to equip God's daughters spiritually, physically, mentally, emotionally, intellectually, and vocationally, to include that sense of "sparkle" that George described? Living God's Divine Wellness Plan for me transitioned me from an unhealthy, unbalanced, egocentric person into a woman who is living a healthy Christ-centered lifestyle. Might my personal testimony on my own experience be able to be heard in the lives of other women? How could these foundations make sense for women who did not have the privilege of theological studies? This journey began for me with my own personal foundations of faith and experience.

Personal Foundation

From childhood through adulthood, I noticed destructive patterns that impacted African American women within the various areas of their lives. Their lack of comprehension on how to integrate biblical truths into their physical lifestyles was apparent as well.

Living a holistic lifestyle for Christ and educating others on how to live in healthy ways has always been my passion. As I ministered to women within my family, profession and community, I noticed their lack of wellness knowledge and their ongoing spiritual and physical lifestyle choices that were not healthy. These women often informed me that their self-identity, self-esteem, and self-worth were rooted in their on-going lifestyle choices. They suggested that their choices resulted from either their negative self-opinions or the damaging reminders by family members of their past mistakes. These women confessed that their crises of identity often revolved around experiences of homelessness, prison time, physical and mental abuse, and single parenting.

It also appeared to me that many African American women accepted the religious traditions of their families without question. They repeated their ancestors' destructive verbal declarations, ate the same unhealthy food, and lived sedentary lifestyles. Many African American women also seemed to accept society's labels (appearance, living conditions, education level, and financial status) which led to low self-esteem, even though God's word affirmed every individual's self-worth. This faulty view of self resulted in religious practices that produced negative fruit in regards to wellness and wholeness, rather than fruit that resulted from walking in faith and victory in Christ. I also observed African American women and their lack of biblical insight on how to live healthy lives within a stressful environment.

My passion and love for these struggling women energized me to step out in faith and help them to walk within God's divine wellness plan. I prayerfully sought the Lord on how to initiate His wellness plan for African American women; yet at the same time, a number of years before this project, I stepped out within my own energy and strength and developed my preconceived wellness plan. While my wellness plan incorporated a daily exercise routine, limited intake of junk food, daily routine prayers, and weekly journaling of mood swings, the results were horrifying. Despite my efforts, the participants continued to lack self-confidence and continuously questioned their decisions.

I went back to God in prayer, searched my heart, and repented for trying to serve others within my own strength. After much soul-searching, the Lord led me through twenty years of preparation within a holistic journey that incorporated various wellness components. A spiritual perspective of my impact on my own and other's spiritual journeys led me into a practice of the discipline of solitude. The time spent in ongoing meditation and the study of God's word began to impact my personal wellness choices. This spiritual discipline led me to incorporate the practice of an evening spiritual check list, leading to soul-searching and self-examination of my words, actions, and thoughts. This was painful at times; however, it was needed to position myself for spiritual growth. It helped me to know God's holistic plan for myself so that I could help others in a way that glorified the Messiah.

Through the guidance of the Holy Spirit, my spiritual growth prompted me to seek educational wellness resources by finding mentors, obtaining degrees (bachelor, master, doctorate), and becoming certified as an aerobic group instructor and personal trainer, as well as a coach for nutrition, health promotions, and basic life support. I enhanced my public speaking skills through Toastmaster International, where I earned the Distinguished Toastmaster certification. My quest to seek more of God in the area of wellness led me to enroll in the Doctor of Ministry degree program at Ashland Theological Seminary. Within the Independent Design track, I focused on the area of wellness. Dr. Matthew Bevere, my initial D. Min. advisor, suggested I incorporate spiritual formation as well as pastoral counseling and care courses. This helped me develop the soul wellness sessions for self and others.

This Bible-based educational program has expanded my knowledge of spiritual wellness and helped me on my journey as a woman of character (Proverbs 31:10-31). It has enhanced my walk of love and service as I denied self-ego (Wardle 2016, 4). Now, my life is alive in Christ as I continued to operate from the fruit of the Spirit: love, joy, peace, forbearance, kindness, goodness, faithfulness, gentleness, and longsuffering (Col. 3:1-17 and Gal. 5:22-23).

Biblical Foundation

Concepts for God's holistic plan for women are found throughout the Old and New Testament. The ultimate prescription for the Christian woman in both spiritual and physical health is that she should mimic the life of the Messiah (Simundson 1982, 331), and passages in both Proverbs and Colossians provide a framework for health and well-being.

The Old Testament passage used in this project, Proverbs 31:24-31, provides a holistic guide for healthy living. This passage was seen not with the goal of perfecting the character traits of virtuous women; instead, the biblical outline can be seen to encourage and motivate Christian women.

The acrostic poem of Proverbs 31 offered God's principles for a successful, healthy lifestyle for single and married women (Branch 2012, 1). John Hartley explained that an understanding of Proverbs 31 provides the tools that women can incorporate into their management skills, their professional careers, and their households (Hartley 2016, 330). The principles found within this chapter can be used for long-term change as they are implemented through women's lifestyles as they reverence Yahweh. Also, a woman can understand that her self-value stems from her trust and reverence in God versus self-pride, physical appearance, or self-deceptive-charm (Hartley 2016, 334). Monica Coleman expressed how this Scripture passage revealed that holistic, disciplined lifestyles were rooted upon their spiritual foundation in God (Coleman 2008, 140).

Transitioning from the Old Testament into the New Testament, the Apostle Paul's letter to the Colossians educated and encouraged his readers to maintain their virtuous lifestyles regardless of their circumstances through grateful hearts, peaceful souls, and forgiving spirits (Col. 3: 1-17). Paul's letter informed his readers that for them to live in a holy way, they must follow the holistic rules for living found within Colossians 3:1-17. Paul's writing encouraged the Christians to die to their earthly nature (old self) and to be "made alive in Christ" (Carson 1991, 500; Col. 3:5-10). The biblical perspective of living as being made alive in Christ, was rooted upon their belief, trust, and obedience to God's word. John Carmody and George Edmond Smith concurred that Paul's letter encouraged the Christians to make their life choices based on their spiritual understanding and intimate relationship with Yahweh (Carmody 1983, 9; Smith 2015, 54). The holistic rules for living within this passage instructed Paul's readers on how to be raised with Christ within their minds, how to "put to death" the works of the flesh, and how to selflessly serve others with compassion, kindness, and patience (Von Speyr, 1998, 123; Weems 1988, 95).

Through this passage, the Christians' awareness of their faith walk in Christ was the spiritual antidote used to help them turn away from coveting the unhealthy lifestyles of others (Col. 3:5-7). Paul's moral teaching exposed the consequences of living outside of God's wellness atmosphere in relation to his readers' lifestyle choices and spoken words (Von Speyr 1998, 118; Martin 1973 113). Paul's letter encouraged the followers of Christ to surrender their old natures (self-will) in order to walk in their new natures as they trust in God's grace.

The next section of the dissertation moves from the pages of Scripture to explore concepts of personhood from a theological perspective.

Theological Foundation

In the realm of theology, a number of topics have impact upon African American women and their understanding of self. The theological basis of the creation of African American women, and the theology of purpose, particularly for women, are considered within the unhealthy (Anthropology) and healthy (Pauline Anthropology) framework. The Pauline Anthropology emphasizes how the harmony between spirit, soul, and body is vital, and addresses the topic of freedom of choice in the areas of health and fitness.

Writers from a womanist perspective were especially helpful, as they reflected upon the health and lifestyles of African American women within their society, even when faced with humiliation, inadequate education, poverty, and enslavement to white labor (Coleman 2008, 336; Floyd-Thomas 2006, 116; Weems, 1988, 17). For example, Monica Coleman argues how the African American woman's intimate relationship with God assisted her through her lifestyle struggles, helping her to overcome oppressions through racism, sexism, and classism (Coleman 2008, 13).

In exploring womanist theology, Mitchem suggests that God created a woman to be a bearer and nurturer of life through childbearing, being, providing beauty (appearance), and offering grace by serving family members and communities (Mitchem 2002, 24). Mitchem wrote that a part of the African American women's self-identity is found within their personal belief and their families' inheritance within society (Mitchem 2002, 24). According to Mitchem, a health and wellness balance for African American women (physiologically, emotionally, mentally, and spiritually) rested upon their ability to accept and operate within God's unique design for them (Mitchem 2002, 5). Yet, often African American women allowed life's complications to determine their wellness choices. This caused an unhealthy balance, which resulted in unhealthy lifestyle choices (Anthropology).

This impact workshop also incorporated Moltmann and Moltann's view that a woman represented "God the Mother" (Moltmann and Moltmann 1991, 38). Their reflections revealed how women were created with the rebirthing power, shared earthly dominion with men, and were helpmates to their spouses (Gen. 2:18).

As in the Old Testament anthropology approach, Bultmann expressed that mankind was a victim of his own ego and self-willed action which caused the death of his being and soul (Moltmann 1985, 259). Moltmann explained that whenever humankind made decisions from their sinful nature, the choices resulted in emotional (soul) decisions, thus causing disharmony between the body, known as *soma,* and soul (Moltmann 1985, 260). Schwarz and McConville concurred that when humans followed the Old Testament anthropology approach, their lifestyles lacked unity within their spirit, soul, and body (Schwarz 2013, 6, 362; McConville 2016, 48).

A further view is that humans were created to love and serve God within a holistic lifestyle that unified soul, spirit, and body. This wholeness of person is known as the Tripartite Anthropology (McConville 2016, 189; Schwarz 2014, 14). This trichotomous viewpoint revealed that when individuals lived holistically, their subsequent health choices coincided with God's wellness plan, also known as Pauline Anthropology (Green 2008, 68).

Ongoing self-identity issues can cause a battle between spirit, soul, and body. In contrast, unity between the spirit, soul, and body (Pauline Anthropology) brings health through God's wholeness plan. This constituted God's truth within a realistic world, beauty through self-acceptance, and peace through making healthy choices (Green 2008, 5; Schwarz 2013, 160; Coleman 2008, 65). Hans Schwarz stated that according to Apostle Paul, the balanced lifestyles for believers were rooted upon their selective health choices to love God with their hearts, strengths and souls in unity (Schwarz 2013, 6).

Historical Foundation

The religious beliefs of African American women often stemmed from their generational faith practices. Their healing methods, deliverance from sinful behaviors, and the overcoming of pain and suffering were possible through their traditional hope, trust, and faith in their cultural belief system. The historical section outlines how the lifestyles of African American women were impacted by the following time periods: Antebellum Era (1812-1861), American Civil War and beyond (1861-1890), and the Twentieth Century (1890-present).

The Antebellum Era, the years from the War of 1812 to the Civil War, revealed how the personal health, hygiene, self-esteem, self-worth, and medical needs of African American women transitioned from self-ownership to slave master's ownership (negative care) (Mitchem 2007, 52; Patterson 2000, 41). The deterioration of the health of African American women resulted from rape by their slave masters, unhealthy living conditions, isolation from family members, and the victimization of slave labor (Patterson 2000, 37; Tannenbaum 2012, 32).

With the Civil War and its aftermath, the health care fears of the African American women became a reality. Medical care for themselves and their family members was classified as "unequal treatment" (White 2011, 211). Medical attention was available for the purpose of research testing, medical experiments, and exploitations (McCloud and Ebron 2003, 5; Golubic 2016, interview). During the Jim Crow era (post-Civil War), the medical treatments received by African American women from some of the Caucasian medical doctors resembled the negative health services they received during slavery. This led them to fear and doubt their health diagnoses, medical prescriptions, and physicians' referrals (White 2011, 212; Washington 2008, 54).

In 1865, the War Department created the Freedmen's Bureau. This allowed freed slaves to receive help with overcoming the challenges of emancipation, particularly those that were social, economic, educational, political and medical (Downs 2012, 45). The freed slaves and African American veterans received temporary shelter, food supplies, clothes and undeveloped medical treatments through Freedom hospitals (Downs 2012, 87). Yet, the federal government denied payment responsibility for the freed African Americans' health care expenses. The African American elite society implemented various benevolence organizations to provide healthcare plans to deal with the war's medical crisis and discriminative labor laws, and to make educational tools available (Downs 2012, 112; Long 2012, 66; Forbes 1998, 165). As the African American women transitioned into the twentieth century, developing and maintaining holistic lifestyles became more promising.

When the United States passed the Civil Rights Act in 1964, one of its goals was to eliminate the racial barriers within the health care system (Thomas 2011,

278). Yet thirty years later, advocates Dula and Goering proclaimed that the treatment available for African American women within the United States remained unfair in relation to services and fees (Dula and Goering 1994). The African American women transitioned from slave entrapments into lifestyles which produced negative stressors and unhealthy holistic balances within their wellness components: physical, mental, emotional, and spiritual (Downs 2012, 43).

In the twentieth century, African American women continued to face stressful racial barriers within medical access and career industries while trying to maintain holistic lifestyles (Lowe 2006, 29). An African American woman's self-worth suffered an identity crisis as she lived within an unhealthy, crowded environment. African American women lacked the educational and professional knowledge to maintain healthy lifestyles in the areas of medical and dental coverage, job security, and family unity (Byrd and Clayton 2000, 215). Their concern for the healthcare plans and career opportunities for themselves, their families, and their communities led them to become healthcare adversaries known as racial up-lifters (Shakir 2016, Lecture).

In this role, African American women became professional educators. They offered health and wellness courses to their family members and neighbors in the areas of hygiene, nutrition, physical health care, mental health care, and lifestyle grief recovery. Workshops on cultural heritage and self-identity in Christ were offered to encourage and motivate the African American women through their life struggles with and within a dominant white society (Mitchem 2004, 129, Johnson 1998, 111). Workshops on true-self-Identity, anchored in Bible-based proclamations, taught acceptance of their self-worth and self-respect in spite of racism, income suppression and discrimination from politicians and inferior medical plans (Johnson, Pitre and Johnson 2014, 123; Katzman 1973, 206).

"Who am I?" was the self-identity question that the African American women pondered and searched, finding peace within their acceptance and recognition of their individual unique womanist identity in Christ (Weems 1988, 94; Cornish 2002, 91). The "whole person" plan, which was rooted in God's wellness plan, delivered the African American women from deceptive thoughts and lifestyles placed upon them through slave trade, generational curses, racism, income suppression, and discrimination from white supremacy (Mitchem 2007, 51; Hull, Scott, and Smith 1982, 250). The African American woman's holistic lifestyle was rooted throughout her family's religious beliefs and interaction with each other in spite of their ongoing negative circumstances.

The contemporary section as noted in Chapter Three examined how advocacies concerning wellness information for African American women benefited the women's personal and professional holistic lifestyles (Johnson, Pitre, and Johnson 2014, 148).

I honor the women of my race. Their beauty, -- their dark and mysterious Beauty of midnight eyes, crumpled hair, and soft, full featured faces – is perhaps more to me than to you because I was born to its warm subtle spell; but their worth is yours as well as mine. No other women on earth could have emerged from hell of force and temptation which once engulfed and still surrounds black women in America with half the modesty and womanliness that they retain. I have always felt like bowing myself before them in all abasement, searching to bring some tribute to these long-suffering victims, these burdened sisters of mine, whom the world, the wise, white world, loves to affront and ridicule and wantonly to insult. I have known the women of many lands and nations, -- I have known and seen and lived beside them, but none have I known more sweetly feminine, more unswervingly loyal, more desperately earnest, and more instinctively pure in body and in soul than the daughters of my black mothers. (W.E.B. Du Bois, Smith 2015, 165)

The contemporary foundation reveals how African American women maintain peace and unity within their spirits, souls and bodies. African American women who rely on their faith to uplift them "through all of the degradation heaped upon them" remain "pure in their body and soul" (Smith 2015, 165). Their faith assisted them in overcoming the negative thoughts instilled in them through the degrading claims of society that states that "nothing decent in womanhood came from black slavery but adultery and uncleanness" (Smith 2015, 165).

These African American women lived within a fast-paced society (the natural world) while maintaining their faith walk (the supernatural world) and healthy lifestyle balance. The dimensions of wellness will address the following three components for holistic living: spirit (relationship with God), soul (mind frame and emotional state), and body (healthcare and self-care).

African American women of faith were able to maintain their spirituality within contemporary society. Their health and wellbeing were rooted upon their ongoing personal relationship with the Messiah and their self-acceptance of their Christ-like identity (Foster 2008, 44). The true identity of the African American women rested within their ongoing self-development in Christ (Benner 2012, 15). Their daily interactions produced Bible-based fruit of the Spirit when they accepted, committed, and followed God's wellness blueprint (Peterson 2006, 23). Womanist writers demonstrated how the various female Bible characters reassured the African American women of God's mercy and grace during times of persecution, exploitation, oppression, and health challenges (Weems 1988, 93).

In the area of the soul, defined here as the emotional and mental health components of a woman's life, the emotional and mental well-being of African American women was negatively impacted historically through ongoing practices of "ism" which destroyed their self-worth, intellectual abilities, and emotional states (Carter and Parker 1996, 248). In both positive and negative ways, their consciousness of their thought patterns revealed the health condition of their frames of mind and emotional states in relation to their self-images (Wardle 2001, 179). Aa one example of an avenue of healing for the soul, the African American woman who responded to the "what if" syndrome by using Dr. Neal-Barnett's psychology healthy mind tips, overcame the fear of failures being exposed, dealing with job discrimination, being a single parent, and having babies out of wedlock (Neal-Barnett 2003, 64).

Misconception and wrongful responsibilities and labels assigned to African American women by others, such as their slave owners, Caucasians, and media representatives, no longer needed to affect their wellbeing, emotional health, physical fitness, and spiritual growth (Villarosa 1994, 367). As they participated in faith-based programs of self-development, African American women were able to maintain their lifestyle balance and wellbeing as they transitioned through the following roles within their daily schedules: wives, daughters, administrators, ministers, elders, entrepreneurs, civil rights activists, and artists (Villarosa 1994, 371). Being aware of their identity in Christ brought stress relief for African American women, and delivered them from feelings of failures in marital issues, poverty status, overlooked job promotions, and classification as uneducated women (Hooks 2015, 19).

Engagement within stress relief sessions can eliminate the pressure from tension brought on through seen and unseen circumstances. This approach equipped the African American women with a stress-reduction strategy to combat threats and attacks against their "whole person" holistic lifestyles (Villarosa 1994, 372; Derosis 1998, 68).

As African American women grew in spirit and soul, they also were no longer willing to accept society's descriptions of their body images, often stereotyped as being overweight, with body shapes described as curvy and with a wide frame. The African American women's body mass index (BMI) does not conform to the "white society's ideal body weight" and dress sizes (Hoytt and Beard 2012, 255; Villarosa 1994, 5).

In contrast to those stereotypes, African American women can accept their Messiah's gracious and loving expression of their physical beauty. Now the question that the African American women ask themselves daily was "How do I take care of myself"? In the late twentieth and now in the twenty-first century, African American women are engaging in health care through self-investments such as saving and investment, me-time, life insurances and burial policies, annual physical checkup, and ongoing educational courses. They also became better educated on how to take care of their unique hair texture, skin tones, body shapes, nutrition, and dress styles suitable for their body composition (McCloud and Ebron 2003, 35; Taylor 2003, 561; Byrd and Solomon 2005, 215; Jack 2010, 29).

The next section will provide information about the project workshops. Also, it will briefly inform the reader of the profiles of the participants.

Context

This project was undertaken in Union-Miles, a low income, primarily black neighborhood on the east side of Cleveland. Many African American women in this neighborhood deal with various past life challenges such as unemployment, homelessness, sexual abuse, addictions, and domestic violence, as well as current life crises. The material used, the Diva's Lifestyle Identity Journey, was designed to instill within the African American women the hope of overcoming past challenges in order to live successfully within their communities.

Weekly holistic group sessions were conducted for six weeks with a group of ten women. Their ages ranged from eighteen to eighty years old. Their career choices varied, and they had different cultural values and family traditions. Two were retired, two were financial accountants, one was a professional hair stylist, one an artist, one a community leader, one a volunteer youth teacher, one a civil rights activist, and one a pastor.

These African American women were women of the Christian faith who volunteered in various capacity within their church, as members of production teams, as worship leaders, trustees, Sunday school teachers, greeters, ushers, and support groups. They all believed that Jesus was their Savior; however, they lacked endurance and strength in the area of living within God's divine wellness plan for them. The participants were selected on a first come first served basis through an online and phone-in registration.

Project Goals

The purpose of this project was to impact the healthcare of women within the Union-Miles community in Cleveland, Ohio by providing six weeks of holistic workshops that help participants integrate God's Divine Wellness plan into their daily lives. This section includes goals related to the project:

1. To impact the participants' personal lifestyle through obedience to God's word.

2. To impact the participants' personal lifestyle through exercise.

3. To impact the participants' personal lifestyle through food nourishment.

4. To impact the participants' personal lifestyle through stress management.

5. To impact the participants' personal lifestyle through their relationships.

6. To impact the participants' personal lifestyle through soul-searching.

Design, Procedure, and Assessment

This impact project was designed as a wellness educational experience to motivate, encourage, and instruct the ten African American women participants on how to incorporate God's wellness plan into their daily lifestyles in the areas of spirit, soul, and body. The research question was: What impact will this six weeks of holistic workshops have on the healthcare of the women within the Union-Miles community in Cleveland Ohio?

For six consecutive weeks for three hours on a Saturday morning, the group engaged in interactive holistic workshops designed by the researcher. Each session incorporated ten minutes for meditation, five minutes for prayer, three minutes for devotional readings, and one minute for reciting the Diva's proclamation. Most of the session content was given by a facilitator who instructed the participants on God's wellness plan for them. Each week one of the following wellness topics was discussed: Stress Release, Identity Crisis, Healthy Heart/Soul, Body Image, Spiritual Check-up, and Healthy Mind. The sessions ended with prayer and creative movements to the theme song *I Know Who I Am* by Sinach.

Weekly blogs offering ongoing moral support through words of encouragement and prayers were posted on the Diva's Lifestyle Identity Journey Facebook account. Also, this Facebook page posted weekly educational tips for exercises, nutrition, spiritual growth, breathing techniques, career support, and financial information. After each class session, the facilitator posted notes within each person's journal in relation to the person's wellness area of concern. Through email, the facilitator sent them weekly updates on their progress, answered personal questions, and shared personal prayers. The quantitative and qualitative pre-test and post-test assessment determined the extent of the impact the interactive workshops had on the participants' lifestyles.

Personal Goals

I believed that God's mercy and grace would permit me to utilize my personal wellness lifestyle, my holistic health expertise, and my marketing and administrative skills to develop health and wellness interactive workshops. I realized that the success of the project rested upon my knowledge of who I am in Christ. Therefore, it was important that I maintain a healthy lifestyle. My personal goals were as follows:

1. To make a greater impact in my spiritual life through intensive integration of spiritual and physical disciplines.

2. To develop a closer relationship with God through intimate relationship with Him.

3. To intentionally accept people's choices when I do not agree with them.

4. To make sure to accept others' viewpoints.

Definition of Terms

African American Health Culture. Their belief about health and disease. See a connection between spirituality, acceptable social behavior, and physical health (Tannenbaum 2012, 8).

Crisis. Circumstances which led participants to attend the Union-Miles free community outreach project (e.g., drug or alcohol recovery, sexual abuse deliverance, financial hardship, domestic violence shelter, and father absenteeism).

God's Divine Wellness Plan. A plan that permits one to engage in daily activities as one operates within a spiritual and physical discipline connection (Martin 1973, 128; Col. 3:1-17).

Holistic Spirituality. The person's spirit, soul, and body are one. The past, present, and future are one "now" (Afrika 2004, 269).

Holistic Lifestyle. A person's lifestyle choices, decisions, and responsibilities that are based upon the person's religious outlook (Carmody 1983, 3).

Human Person. It unifies the three-distinct unity, body, spirit and soul.

Slavocracy. Term used to correspond with slave owners (merchants, brokers and planters) who were "speculators in slave disposal, who acquired ownership of slaves and plantations by fair or foul means" (Thompson 1987, 131).

Wholeness Lifestyle. A term used to describe a unifying lifestyle. God's wellness plan permits His people to worship and serve Him with physical fitness, body, mind and soul (3 John 1:2 paraphrase).

Woman of Character. A woman whose lifestyle reveals and reverences the wisdom of God (Koptak 2003, 674).

Womanism. A post-colonial discourse that allows African American women to embrace a Jesus and a God free of the imperialism of white supremacy (Weems 1988, 82; Mitchem 2002, 122).

Womanist Theology. A term that defines and describes the African American woman's theological perspective as rooted upon her faith during her life circumstances, family traditions, church teaching, system of ethics, and challenge ecclesiastical structures (Mitchem 2002, 60).

Plan of the Paper

This chapter has introduced the structure for the research approach for this impact project. The following chapters will include biblical, historical, and theological foundations (Chapter Two); a review of contemporary literature (Chapter Three); a detailed description of the method, procedures, and design of the project (Chapter Four); and the results of the project (Chapter Five). The final chapter will reflect on the impact of the project goals and my personal goals, and will consider their application to ministry as well as the potential for further study (Chapter Six).

CHAPTER TWO

BIBLICAL, THEOLOGICAL AND HISTORICAL FOUNDATIONS

It is important for the Christian female to know that her inward and outward beauty glorifies her creator, *Elohim*, since she is "fearfully and wonderfully made" (Psalm 139:14 NIV). (All scripture references will be from the NIV unless otherwise noted). *El-Elyon*, the Highest God, created all people to worship Him. God assigned women the responsibility of assisting their husbands, children, co-workers, and communities by practicing servant leadership (Branch 2012, 9).

God's love for woman is revealed through His acceptance and appreciation of her uniqueness in body and character. In response, women illustrate their love for God through their service to others within their households, their industries, and throughout their daily activities. The focus of this chapter is to explore the foundations for this project. The three foundations will be addressed in the following order: biblical, theological, and historical.

Biblical Foundation

There are special parts of ourselves that play a critical role in health and healing. Listen to your heart, for it's in your heart where the feelings tell you, "I'm not quite complete, not quite where I want to be," Once you hear that, honor it. Then you can begin to do something. (Dr. Marcellus A. Walker cited by McCloud and Ebron 2003,32)

The Old and New Testaments identify a woman's character, behavior, and role within her household and community (Simundson 1982, 331). God's wellness plan encourages women to worship and serve Him wholeheartedly: spirit, soul, and body (3 John 1:2). God's word motivates and encourages women after God's own heart to identify, accept, and mimic His character throughout their daily lives. In this chapter, a passage from Proverbs 31:24-31 will be studied as it reflects the attributes of a woman of virtue. In the New Testament passage, the topic of holistic rules for holy living will be explored within the context of Christian behavior in the third chapter of Colossians.

Proverbs 31:24-31

As background to this passage, the words of Proverbs 31 form the concluding chapter in this book of collected wisdom, as the writer describes his poetic image of a wise woman, a woman of valor. The poem structure used by the author is an acrostic. Starting with the first letter of the Hebrew alphabet, it follows in sequence through the rest of the alphabet, as its stanzas outline a woman of strength and describe her value to others (Fox 2009, 891). The acrostic poem reflects a woman of worth who is a skilled wife within an early Jewish household.

The Hebrew poet appears to have a two-fold goal in writing Proverbs 31. First, in verses 1-9, the writer offers a message to Lemuel from his mother, addressing how to gain wisdom for living, and warning of the need to avoid promiscuous women and drunkenness (Fox 2009, 890). As a second purpose, the poet uses verses 10-31 to provide a visual illustration of a woman of strength.

The acrostic poem identifies a woman as being of noble character, diligent, caring, and wise. She displays moral worth within her household. As Joel Biwul notes, her "fear of Yahweh" is the foundation for her moral worthiness and godliness (Biwul 2013, 281). Her active role within this large household is to implement her managerial skills while exemplifying the following characteristics: strength, independence, courage, kindness, wisdom and piety, as her relationship with God helps her to serve her family and the members of society (Biwul 2013, 282).

The word used to describe this woman is found within the first verse of this section of the chapter, often referred to as the epilogue, when the writer asks, "A wife of noble character; Who can find?" (v. 10). The term, translated in the NIV as noble character, is *esheth khayil*. *Khayil* is a common term in the Old Testament, described by Hermann Eising in this way: "Despite the frequent occurrence of *khayil* in the sense of 'army,' its basic meaning must be given as 'strength, power' (Eising 1980, 348). Other translations for *esheth-khayil* include the following: "virtuous woman" (KJV), "excellent wife" (NAS), "valiant woman" (DRA) and "worthy wife" (NAB). Other translations use "excellent" (ESV), "capable" (NJB, NRS), and "virtuous" (NK, NLT) (Biwul 2013, 281). Megan DeFranza suggests that the translation of this word "should retain the primary sense of khayil as 'strength,'" in order to "convey the primary meaning of the Hebrew text; second, to render more carefully the meaning of *khayil* in the context of Proverbs 31; and, last, to overcome the disparate portraits of men and women in the Hebrew Bible" (DeFranza 2001, 18). These translations of *esheth-khayil* will be used interchangeably in the remainder of this section.

Because this project focused on how to support African American woman as they discovered their own strength within the context of their faith, I chose the specific pericope of Proverbs 31:24-31 as my Old Testament focus. Critical elements in the passage are defined as being a woman of valor, wealth, strength and power. In this section, the characteristic of a woman of strength as a role model will be examined in the following areas: bringing income into her home, speaking kindness and wisdom, caring for her household, and living in fear of God (Branch 2012, 9). Comparisons will also be made to Ruth and the Hebrew midwives, other Old Testament women of strength and courage.

Contributing Income (Proverbs 31:24)

Verse 24 of Proverbs 31 illustrates how this model woman was able to contribute to the financial support of her household. "She makes linen garments and sells them, and supplies the merchants with sashes." This woman of worth visually exhibited her spirit of hard work within her industrious engagements (Biwul 2013,292). As a Jewish housewife and mother, she served with a virtuous care while using her managerial skill to augment her family income. She exemplifies the attributes of an industrious and God-fearing female as she made and sold luxury linen to be worn as outer wrapping (Fox 2009, 896).

Mmapula Diana Kebaneilwe suggests that another biblical woman of industry, strength and courage was Ruth, with similar descriptions to the Proverbs 31 woman (Kebaneilwe 2012, 16). Ruth, like the woman of valor, was loyal to the welfare of her family, in particular Naomi (Ruth 2:1-21). The industriousness of both Ruth and the woman of valor benefit their family as they zealously worked with their hands (Kebaneilwe 2012, 161).

Clothed with Dignity (Proverbs 31:25)

"She is clothed with strength and dignity; she can laugh at the days to come" (31:25). A woman of character reverenced the Lord through her lifestyle while "she is clothed with strength and dignity" (George 2014, 190; Prov. 31:25a). Reading this verse literally, the woman of strength has a dress attire that "befits her status" (Fox 2009, 897), while a figurative reading would reflect her character.

In the second half of verse 25, her confidence, shown through her laughter suggests that she prepares her household for their future needs and for her old age (Prov. 31:25b). As noted in the translations of the term *khayil* used at the beginning of the poem, the woman's roles as wife, mother, and industrial influencer are described by words that visually illustrate her moral worth, ability and strength within her household and within the industry (Biwul 2013, 281). Thus, the woman of worth is a diligent worker, loyal towards others, and, as the next verse reminds the reader, she keeps her word (Prov. 31:26).

Spoken Words (Prov. 31:26)

Proverbs, says Ellen Davis, are "essentially oral literature: they circulate by word of mouth" (Davis 2000,12), so it is no surprise that the woman who concludes the book of Proverbs contributes to her world through spoken word, oral literature. Throughout the book of Proverbs, emphasis has been given to word choices and their end results (Prov.13:2-3; Prov.18: 21; 20:19), and Proverbs 31 begins with

Lemuel's mother expressing her concern about a king's lifestyle choices and his selective choice to marry woman of wisdom (God fearing) versus a woman of folly (promiscuous).

This pattern of the importance of the spoken word as well as the words being spoken by a woman is suggested again in verse 26. This virtuous woman "speaks with wisdom, and faithful instruction is on her tongue" (Prov. 31:26). DeFranza recognizes that the phrase *torah-khesed* (faithful instruction) "is unique. It could refer to her mode of teaching (with the kindness of a mother rather than harshness of a father), teaching modeled on her generosity, or a particular body of instructions, such as the contents of Proverbs" (DeFranza 2011, 19).

The woman of courage exhibits the word choices used within her work and home environment (Kebaneilwe 2012, 158). The woman of wisdom in relation to word choices is a second similarity the woman of valor shares with the biblical character Ruth. Ruth's actions of goodness and kindness toward Naomi and interaction with Boaz revealed words spoken in wisdom. Boaz spoke about Ruth's acts of kindness and goodness towards Naomi and himself (Ruth 2:11; Ruth 3:11).

The woman of worth, of noble character within Proverbs 31 speaks with wisdom as she deals within the community, and when she teaches her children (Fox 2009, 897). Her wise words are reinforced through her actions as her home atmosphere is filled with love, care, and solace (Biwul 2013, 282). During her conversations, she speaks God's word as she judges others with integrity. Her husband uses his own word combination to praise and reveal his confidence for his wife of noble character (Prov. 31:11). Her words spoken to him or about him: "bring him good, not harm all the days of her life" (Prov. 31:12; Biwul 2012, 285).

Family Care

An additional characteristic of the woman of noble character is her trustworthy, noble, faithful, and god-fearing service as she engages in family care (Prov. 31:27). A woman of courage lovingly "watches over the affairs of her household and does not eat the bread of idleness" (Ehlke 1992, 316). She oversees their behavior; therefore, her household activities are not limited to childbearing and mothering. Her domestic role includes nurturing and educating her offspring, being a helper to her spouse, and providing present and future healthcare, food and clothing (Dube 2001, 152). In verse 27, she is concerned with the future care of her loved ones. She spends hours working eagerly with her hands, covering beds, clothing herself with strength and dignity, dressing family members in fine linen, and avoiding idle activities (Ehlke 1992, 317).

Matrimonial faithfulness rested upon her virtuous traits of loyalty and trust as well (Dube 2001, 150; Hartley 2016, 331). As the woman of wisdom meets the needs of family members (Prov. 31:14-15, 21-22), her husband praises her (Prov. 31:28). She received the confidence and trust from her husband who "is respected at the city gate" (Prov. 31:11, 23).

Her service to her family flourishes from her belief in spiritual discipline and God's holiness (Hartley 2016, 333; Prov. 31:25-27). This alphabetic poem illustrates the woman's avoidance of complaining, grumbling, and sulking over being an early riser or speaking words of wisdom (Biwul 2013, 280). Her strength and honor rest within her reverence and fear of the Lord. At home, she tirelessly and selflessly serves her husband and children per their individual desires and needs (George 2014). The service to her family results in her work bringing her praise at the city gate (Prov. 31:31b)

Fear of the Lord

The closing verses of this passage are found in Proverbs 31:29-31. "Many women do noble things, but you surpass them all. Charm is deceptive, and beauty is fleeting, but a woman who fears the Lord is to be praised. Honor her for all that her hands have done, and let her works bring her praise at the city gate." As DeFranka notes, the use of the word *khayil*, the description given to her at the beginning of the poem, is repeated in verse 29 (DeFranka 2011, 19). DeFranka suggests that "the reintroduction of khayil (v. 29) beautifully ties the end of the poem with its opening title. In this verse, it is connected to the woman's action, rather than her person, and renews the connection with the heroic deeds accomplished in military context" (DeFranka 2011, 19).

This is indeed "a woman who fears the Lord" (Prov. 31:30). Her admiration of the Lord results with her using her godly wisdom to assist her family and industry while she earns "honor, respect, and dignity" (Biwul 2013, 294; Prov. 31:30-31). A woman of character knows that her beauty resides in her reverent fear of the Lord and spiritual character, versus the emptiness of charm and physical beauty (Prov. 31:30).

As Whybray notes, "the Fear of Yahweh is a key concept in Proverbs" Whybray 1995, 136). It is first found in Proverbs 1:7, and then its final use is here in Proverbs 31:30, creating "a literary envelope around the book," as it "illustrates the concrete embodiment of theoretical wisdom" (Ansberry 2010, 181).

While the term "fear of the Lord" is used extensively in the book of Proverbs, and in the Old Testament, it is generally not used in a gender-specific way, as in Proverbs 9:10, "The fear of the Lord is the beginning of wisdom." However, it is the same phrase that is used of the Hebrew midwives in Exodus 1:17. Cheryl Exum suggests that this fear of God is "a far broader theological concept, having at its center the element of *mysterium tremendum*, and extending to conduct that is guided by basic ethical principles and in harmony with God's will" (Exum 1994, 62).

21

Just as Ruth is compared to the woman of valor in Proverbs 31, so too can the comparison be made between the woman of valor and the Hebrew midwives, as their "fear of the Lord" informed their actions.

The virtuous woman's recognition of honor is evidenced within her spiritual formation and noble character (Hartley 2016, 330). Her character traits are a part of a continuous development process that revealed her spiritual and physical beauty which glorified God (George 2014, 9). The female's true character (reverencing Yahweh) was seen through her children who praised her for her righteous, moral, noble, and godly character (Biwul 2013, 286).

The crowning virtue for a woman of courage is in her reverent fear of the Lord. The woman of wisdom's strength is found within her adoration for Yahweh. Her godly character is established upon admiration for the Lord. The woman is praised by her children and husband because she fears the Lord.

To conclude this section, a helpful synopsis of this passage is provided by Tremper Longman:

> Another of the dominant themes throughout the poem is the woman's boundless energy. It is hard to believe that any single person could ever accomplish as much as this ideal woman, and perhaps the description is meant as a composite sketch. In any case, this woman is described not only as a warrior but also as a merchant ship that brings produce to port, namely her home. She also is active in commercial endeavors, not to speak of philanthropy toward the needy. Not only are her actions praised, but also her qualities of mind and attitude. She is fearless about the future, wise and kind. This woman has nothing at all to do with laziness. The emphasis at the end of the poem, as one might expect, is not on beauty or charm, but on the woman's fear of the Lord. Indeed, this woman is the epitome of wisdom. She is the human embodiment of God's wisdom; a flesh-and-blood personification of Woman Wisdom. (Longman 2006, 141)

The Proverbs 31:24-31 passage is a description of a woman of noble character, particularly in regards to her actions and reverent fear of the Lord. The woman of strength receives praises and is blessed through her service to others because she fears the Lord. If Proverbs 31 is focused on the actions of the body, the New Testament passage of Colossians 3:1-17 suggests a comparable emphasis on the spirit and soul. In the letter of Paul to the Colossians, both men and women are given direction as to how to live in a holy fashion. The next section will discuss the rules for holy living needed for wellness maintenance as found within Colossians 3:1-17.

Colossians 3:1-17

In his letter to the Colossians, the Apostle Paul urged Christians to live virtuous lifestyles by denying self-righteousness since they were "made alive in Christ" (Carson 1991, 500). The scriptural blueprint found within Colossians 3:1-17 offers holistic rules for holy living which women can use for guidance as they seek a whole and healthy lifestyle. In relation to wellness through behavior, the following three areas will be discussed as reflected in Paul's letter: mindset, works of the flesh, and relationships.

Mindset

As Paul recognized throughout his letters, a person's mindset was essential to a life in Christ. "Set your mind on things above . . ." (Col. 3:2). Intake of God's word focuses one's thought on Christlikeness instead of unproductive malicious thoughts (Whitney 1991, 133).

Paul's letter to the Colossians informed them that they were to be worshippers of God, and not to become students of false doctrine or to become receptors of evil appearances (Barclay 1961, 44). Paul's writing in Col. 3: 16-17 taught his readers that their minds should be rooted in God's word (Wright 2008, 148). William Barclay stated that avoidance of religious syncretism was accomplished from wisdom that the Christians received through meditation on Scripture. Religious syncretism is defined as the fusion of diverse religious beliefs and practices (Barclay 1961, 132). The letter to the Colossians reassured Paul's readers that keeping their mind set on things above kept their lives "hidden with Christ in God" (Col. 3:2-4).

Paul's note offered a refresher course on the importance of a lifestyle that revolved around God's word (Von Speyr 1998, 130; Col. 3:16-17) and the model of the Messiah's authentic earthly ministry (Matt. 4-20; Mark 1-10; Luke 3-19; John 2-11). Avoidance of religious syncretism was accomplished through dwelling and learning God's word joyously which produced His wisdom (Wright 2008, 148). Paul wrote that the actions, choices, and spirituality of the saints should display their Christian virtue and represent the Lord Jesus (Synge 1958, 90).

The letter to the Colossians was written in part to teach the reader that the focal point of the believer's whole life was to worship and praise God, to avoid the appearance of evil, and to steer clear from false doctrine (Barclay 1961, 31-45). Paul wanted to educate the readers on the outcomes of two-paths, one old and the other new (Beetham 2010, 231). The pathway of false teaching resulted in the choice of the old and sinful nature (Gen. 1: 26-27; Gen. 3: 1-13).

Paul's message proclaimed that to be content with the old nature would result in God's wrath (Beetham 2010, 240; Col. 3:6). Obeying the leadership of the pagans led the Colossians to fulfill the lust of the flesh: passions, evil desires, covetousness, and impurities (Martin 1973, 109; Col. 3: 5-8). The letter informed the Christians at Colossae that living in the flesh meant living in an unregenerate lifestyle, the old nature (Bruce 1977, 205; Gal. 5: 19-20; Col. 3: 5-9).

Paul pointed out that they are no longer in bondage to their flesh if the Spirit of Christ dwelt within them (Beetham 2010, 241; Col. 3: 10, 12). The Christian's new nature, the unity between God and the believer, resulted in a restored state of holiness, true righteousness, and a spiritually disciplined lifestyle (Beetham 2010, 242; Gal. 5: 22-25: Col. 3: 10,12-16). Paul's letter expressed how God's love provided them with a new spiritual wardrobe: humility, kindness, love, and forbearance (Wright 2008, 146-148; Martin 1973, 119-127; Col. 3: 11-17).

Works of the Flesh

In order to live as "God's chosen people, holy and dearly loved," the Colossian Christians needed to safeguard themselves against fulfilling the lust of the flesh: sexual immorality, lust, evil desires and greed (Col. 3:5). Paul's writing discussed the "works of the flesh" such as anger attacks, malicious behaviors, and verbal abuse to self and others (Col. 3: 5-9; Gal. 5: 19-21). Paul's letter was the holistic defense used to alert and assist the Christians in knowing and overcoming the temptations to yield their spirits and bodies to habitually lustful acts (Martin 1973, 109;).

Paul's letter addressed how to handle situations that threatened and caused one to abandon one's faith (Barclay 1961, 30). Paul encouraged the Christians to allow their holistic lifestyle to be free from spiritual malnutrition such as greed, jealously, envy and strife. The Apostle commented on how to prevent the human body from engaging in the "works of the flesh": evil desire, covetousness, malice, foul talk, and self-fulfillment of the old nature (Martin 1973, 109; Col. 3:5-9; Gal.5:19–21). Paul's letter proclaimed how spiritual discipline and true self-denial were the antidotes used to defeat the "works of the flesh" (Martin 1973, 108; Col. 3: 5-11).

Paul's writing warned the new Christians of the danger of a covetous, unhealthy lifestyle (Col.3:5-7). The letter to the Colossians encouraged its readers to die to earthly desires and passions which restricted their faith walk in Christ (Von Speyr 1998, 113; Col. 3: 8-11). Idolatry resulted in archetype worship where one is praising God's creations and resulted in a detour in one's lifestyle away from Christ (Von Speyr 1998, 114). Paul's moral teaching inspired Christians to denounce the desire for wealth or the possessions of others by finding comfort in their old nature.

This could be accomplished by walking in their renewed distinctive Christian character or their new nature (Moule 1957, 119).

The apostle's letter, which were written to encourage the Colossians to live for Christ and to avoid evil practices, warned them of the consequences of corrupt communication and malice (Martin 1973, 112; Col. 3:8). God spoke the world into existence and generously gave His creation, humankind, the same authority through their spoken words. Words create an atmosphere of death and life, reveal one's heart, and results in God's blessing or God's righteous anger (Von Speyr 1998, 118; Col. 3:6,8). Paul reminded the Christians at Colossae that their spoken words influenced their ethical decisions. The believers' word choices should therefore reflect their conversion and spiritual renewal in Christ. The new lifestyle in Christ was initiated when the Colossians submitted to the death to flesh (Wright 2008, 138).

Relationships

To help the Christian guard against the implementation of false teaching into their daily activities, Paul listed "distinctive characters of Christian living", which are love, peace, forgiveness, humility, and forbearance (Martin 1973, 120; Col. 3: 12-17). His message consisted of five moral qualities that a saint used when serving others: compassion, kindness, humility, gentleness, and patience, all relational qualities (Martin 1973, 122; Col. 3:12). Paul instructed them that their daily interactions should portray one or more of those values (Martin 1973, 121-122).

Believers who were connected to Christ visually proclaimed that they were living in Christ (Ladd 1974, 494). Paul reminded the Colossians that they were loved by God and chosen to walk in holiness. They were set apart for God's service. Paul exhorted his readers to put on the moral qualities of Christ (Wright 2008, 146; Col. 3: 12).

As a chosen generation, Paul's readers were holy and beloved (Von Speyr 1998, 122). Paul reminded the believers that the mark placed upon them by their creator required them to glorify and mimic their "maker and heavenly Father" (Wright 2008, 145). The letter noted that a Christian's intimacy with Christ was vividly revealed through the believer's humble services and deeds of kindness (Barclay 1961,126).

The apostle also instructed the citizens of Colossae to interact with each other in the spirit of tolerance and forgiveness (Col. 3:13). Being a realist, Paul stated that the human response to others' weaknesses, bad habits, or false accusations should be based upon God's forgiving plan of redemption (Von Speyr 1998, 125). In doing so, Paul accentuated the importance of restraining one's personal opinions and natural reactions toward others' actions or responses about situations or circumstances (Wright 2008, 146).

Paul reminded the Colossian Christians that walking in love overruled bitterness, anger and unforgiveness (Martin 1973, 119; Col. 3: 14). This Jewish writer, Paul, stressed that choosing to walk in His love manifested their belief in the all-sufficient Christ and detoured them from engaging in the "Colossian heresy" (Barclay 1961,45). The Colossian heresy, false teaching and malpractice, had invaded the churches in Rome and Philippi. It had rapidly entered the spiritual teaching within the Colossian churches (Bruce 1977, 412). The Colossian heresy consisted of a mix of Judaism and the Greek philosophy of Gnosticism (Bruce 1977, 413). Paul condemned the Colossian heresy since its practice detoured the Colossians from God's word of wisdom, knowledge and love walk (Bruce 1977, 417). Paul proclaimed that relationships and daily choices without love were distorted and lacked unity and peace (Wright 2008, 147).

The letter to the Colossians encouraged God's followers to love others and live a peaceful life (Col. 3:15). Living in the peace of Christ unified the believer's soul and body (Synge 1958, 90). Peace within themselves and among others was essential for their spiritual growth and for maintaining healthy relationships within their communities. The "peace of Christ" (v.15) characterized the church community as one body, incorporated a lifestyle of wholeness, purified heart and physical health, and impacted its environment (Wright 2008, 148).

In Proverbs 31, God provided a template for the women of the Old Testament on which to model their lifestyles as they engaged in their daily activities. Healthy lifestyle instructions for Christ-followers in the New Testament were recorded within the Apostle Paul's letters to the Colossians regarding how to live for Christ (Von Speyr 1998, 132). The visual, Bible-based instructions within the Colossian letter educated the Colossians on how to make healthy decisions which would develop and maintain a wellness lifestyle (spiritual, soul, and body) that glorified God. In the following section, a woman who focuses on God's dignity and equality during her wellness journey will be viewed from a theological perspective.

Theological Foundation

Where sin abounded, grace has abounded the more: that is the holistic Christian's main slogan. The love of God at the center of Jesus' preaching and person is at least latent in all the dimensions of human living. We go into no dimension unpreceded by God, need consider none foreign or hostile. Still the practical question remains: How can I boil this down, compact and point it, to start making holism a pattern of daily living? (John Carmody 1983, 3)

In the first section of this chapter, the biblical portrayal of a woman's wellness life-cycle was based upon her spiritual understanding and intimate relationship with

God (Kanyoro 202,3). The theological foundation will explore the theology of creation and the implications for women. The divine purpose for women will be viewed through the anthropology of the Apostle Paul who sees a balance between spirit, soul, and body. This is foundational for understanding the freedom of women to make good choices regarding their health.

Often, the African American woman lived within a negative environment, influenced by society's oppressions and hypocrisy due to their skin color, and deprivation through economic, political, and social rights (Thurman 1996, 53). Regardless of their various known and unforeseen circumstances, African American women were and are able to overcome these circumstances because of their inner strength which resided in their mindfulness of God's Holy Spirit within. Remembering Bible stories and drawing upon their personal faith in Christ helped sustain them as well (Thurman 1996, 102). African American women's self-identity crisis revolved around their daily interactions with others and daily self-treatments through their freedom of choice. Thus, the theological underpinnings that include a balanced walk of faith, acknowledging their purpose and the role of body, soul and spirit were important factors in the development of a healthy lifestyle.

Woman's Purpose

The biblical perspective of humanity is portrayed in Genesis1, the chapter of universal construction (Green 2008, 61; Gen. 1:26-31). The breath of life, imparted from God into the human, resulted in the human becoming a living being. *Nefesh hayah* in Hebrew means "living being" (Schwarz 2013, 6). Lisa Sowle Cahill wrote that the woman's destiny came from her place as Adam's companion, originating from the man himself (Cahill 1992, 25). This male and female relationship provided their earthly purposes: the unity of the flesh, filling the earth with their kind, and sharing in the stewardship responsibilities over other earthly creations (Cahill 1992, 25).

The couple received God's divine vocation and were the only part of creation able to directly communicate with their maker, *Elohim*. The existence of the woman and man illustrated a holy behavior, rooted in God's character, providing the man and the woman with family and community (Green 2008, 61). Green vividly expressed that the life-giving breath was for relational purposes with God, self, family, and neighborhood (Green 2008, 65).

Green and Miller defined human interpersonal earthly ministry as a representation of God's glory (Green 2008, 65; Miller 2004,63). The true self-identity of the male and female was rooted in their connection with God, their heavenly counsel (Green 2008, 67). Cahill acknowledged that man and woman were created equal in God's sight; however, the sin Adam and Eve committed in Eden resulted in

God's judgement and the distortion of their nature personally, socially, and cosmically (Cahill 1992, 29). This act of sin initiated sexual hierarchy, separation of roles, women suffering in childbearing, and the submission of the woman to her husband's rule (Cahill 1992, 28). Jürgen Moltmann argued that a woman represented "God the Mother" who was created with rebirthing power and who was to share earthly dominion with Adam (Moltmann and Moltmann 1991).

Mitchem, who speaks from the viewpoint of womanist theology, stated that an African American woman's response to her creation and the life adjustments that she makes was based upon her deep roots within her biblical beliefs and her personal and family inheritance. An African American female's viewpoint towards her lifestyle stemmed from her essentialist thinking about her universal role and placement between God's Word and society's standards (Mitchem 2002,24, 5). Social gender entrapment placed a woman of color in poverty, inadequate education, and enslavement to white labor (Sanders 1995, 107). Yet God's self-value for all women was equality under His forgiveness, which incorporated the spiritual self-care plan in the areas of martyrdom, humiliation, oppression, income stature, and living conditions (Mitchem 2002, 9).

Humanity's misuse of God's gift of free will has interfered with the unity between spirit, soul, and body within God's creation. The ongoing battles between health and sickness have caused a division among a person's soul and body. This is known as the Anthropology theory (Old Testament). God's Salvation Plan, also known as Pauline Anthropology (New Testament), reestablished unity and harmony within the relationship between men and women and within their holistic journey (Schwarz 2013, 270; Mitchem 2002, 41; Green 2008, 106). A creative wellness plan for humans encourages a person to engage in an ongoing process of self-identity and wellness, a journey toward wholeness that engages spirit, soul, and body (Elwell 2001, 732; Green 2008, 18).

Anthropology

Old Testament theologians Green and Elwell focused on humanity's sinful nature and the dual relationship between nature and God, an anthropology theory (Green 2008, 8; Elwell 2001, 730). Rudolf Bultmann asserted that human existence was based upon the body, *"soma"* (Bultmann 1951,194). George Ladd expressed that humans were a victim to the flesh and sinful nature (Ladd 1974, 471).

Moltmann stated that the body and soul functioned as a fragmentary union (Moltmann 1985, 260). The *soma, or* body, has its own language and memory which was different from the soul's conscious recollection (Moltmann 1985, 260;). Various diverse responses between verbal language and body language assumed an equivocation between soul (inward) and body(outward) (Moltmann 1985, 261). In

God in Creation, man's body, Adam, was formed from earth and was similar to animals. They shared a living soul, living space, eating food, and reproduction for survival (Moltmann 1985, 188). On earth, the body overrode the soul. Humankind was created to physically represent God within the universe (Moltmann 1985, 215).

Schwarz expands the body and soul conversation, explaining that the Old Testament described human beings in four separate Hebrew terms: *nefesh, baser, ruah,* and *leb* (Schwarz 2013, 5-12), essential components of the human being. Integration of *nefesh, baser, ruah,* and *leb* was not necessary, since one's daily activities were based upon the main human need during that time: soul, flesh, spirit, and heart (Schwarz 2103, 13). Individual responses for human survival were based upon the requirement for the human's in-the-moment self-assessment versus the need for a healthy harmonious relationship between *nefesh*, "the soul," *baser,* "the flesh," *ruah,* "the spirit," *and leb* "the heart" (Schwarz 2013,45). If one's living being was emotionally challenged, *nefesh*, the soul, became the focus point for human's survival (Schwarz 2013, 6). Humankind's daily survival alternated between the needs of the body, breath of life (Theo-anthropological), and blood circulation (Schwarz 2013, 382).

McConville concurred with Schwarz's view of the Old Testament language of anthropology. He demonstrated that the complexity of the human holistic lifestyle rested upon being created in the image of God (McConville 2016, 48). The *leb,* "heart," associated with the sinful nature of the inner life, was linked to character and self-importance (McConville 2016, 53; Ps. 101:4; Ezek. 31:10; Deut. 9:5). The book of Deuteronomy emphasized the psychology of nature (McConville 2016, 55). This philosophy identified the intellectual understanding of the "human constitution" of collective and individual interaction of people within the community (McConville 2016, 53; Deut.1: 9-18; 16: 18-17:8).

Pauline Anthropology

Looking at the question of anthropology from a New Testament perspective, humankind was created to love God with a unified soul, heart, and body. This is described as a tripartite anthropology (McConville 2016, 189). This trichotomous viewpoint of man included three distinct components: body, soul, and spirit (Moltmann 1985, 227). In Pauline Anthropology, humankind's personal constituents in relation to God and nature were to be in agreement with the *nefesh, baser,* and *ruah,* (Green 2008, 68).

Pauline Anthropology regarded the human individual as a whole person. The ongoing battle for self-identity between the body, soul, and spirit", the trichotomous, was the understanding within a Pauline Anthropology (Elwell 2001, 732; Green 2008, 5; Schwarz 2013, 160). Schwarz 's study revealed that a believer's daily activities harmoniously rested upon the integration between the spirit, soul, and body (Schwarz 2013, 17). According to Paul, the wholeness of a Christian was rooted upon the believer's love for God with all his or her heart, strength, and soul in unity (Schwarz 2013, 16).

This holistic approach was based on humanity's need for God's divine grace (Elwell 2001, 731; Ladd 1974, 479). The sinful nature (flesh) of humankind, which originated from the first rebellious state of Adam and Eve, was purified through the shed blood of the Lamb, the last Adam, Jesus Christ (Bruce 1977, 330; Green 2008, 99). Human slavery to sin, which diminished a holistic lifestyle, had dominated the choices of the law-abiding citizen (Green 2008, 101; Ladd 1974, 473). Green illustrated how the multidimensional unhealthy lifestyle practices caused war within one's soul and body and resulted in the following sinful living conditions: idolatry, wickedness, rebelliousness, homosexuality, and adultery (Green 2008, 101-105).

The holistic balance between the spirit, soul, and body delivered humankind from the performance trap, operating in sin from one's flesh (Schwarz 2013, 171-173). Pauline Anthropology illustrated how harmony between the spirit and flesh was successful when the believer submitted his or her tripartite being to God's wellness plan (Schwarz 2013, 175). A healthy lifestyle within one's earthly ministry revealed God's lordship. Joe Green, Jurgen Moltmann, and Cheryl Sanders proclaimed that the doctrine of sovereignty, the Son's submission to the Father, was mimicked by a Christian when the saint's spirit ruled over the believer's body (Green 2008, 68; Moltmann 1985, 252; Sanders 1995, 66). The holistic lifestyle within a family environment depended upon each person's freedom of choice to either follow Christ's "spirit" or follow the lust of the person's flesh (body) (Green 2008, 99).

Freedom of Choice

Womanist theologians Sanders and Mitchem concur that African American women, whose holistic lifestyles rest upon their personal relationship and faith in Jesus Christ, did not have to be defeated by either dysfunctional relationships, racism, sexism, or poverty (Sanders 1995, 72; Mitchem 2002,114). For Christian African American women, the visual image of Jesus as co-sufferer provided reassurance that the Messiah struggled along with them and respected their freedom (Coleman 2008, 13). The African American woman's acceptance of Jesus in faith, along with her nurturing from God, motivated and empowered her to confront spiritual death, generational curses, chronic diseases, emotional drama, and vocational discrimination (Mitchem 2002, 122).

Mpyana Fulgence Nyengele states that women's physical health and self-concept suffers from the results of oppression because of their traditional cultural values, as well as from physical and psychological risks (Nyengele 2004, 40). Both

Nyengele and Smith also recognize that sociocultural, religious, and African traditions can restrict and constrain an African American woman's health and wellbeing (Nyengele 2004, 28; Smith 2015, 273). The absence of male-headed families, societal pressures, emphasis on cultural expectations of marriage, lack of education and economic discrimination all contributed to the identity crisis among African American women (Nyengele 2004, 40-50; Amoah1995, 1-7; Oduyoye 2001, 34).

Some of the difficulty that African American women have faced is that Bible readings were used to and will continue to be used "to rationalize the subjugation of African people of the diaspora living in North America including sexual and gender subjugation of African women of the diaspora living in America" (Smith 2015, 48). African American women endured racism, sexism, and classism because they believed that Christ suffered with them (Coleman 2008, 22). Yet is response, Monica Coleman explained how lifestyles which mimicked Jesus maintained wellness and balance including spirit, soul, and body instead of living from the performance trap of operating from self-will (Coleman 2008, 15).

According to Jürgen Moltmann, free will and Christian faith are rooted in "the theology of the cross" (Moltmann and Moltmann 1991, 63). Jesus felt emotional disparity, rejection, and isolation when he prayed in the Garden of Gethsemane; yet, the Messiah obeyed His Father's command and was executed at Golgotha (Moltmann 1991, 65-67). In light of the suffering of Jesus, African American women therefore believed their Savior, Jesus Christ, comforted, suffered, and walked with them through daily adversities and victories (Mitchem 2002, 123; Hollies 2003, 87; Coleman 2008, 13).

Mpyana Fulgence Nygengele, a theologian at the Methodist Theological School in Ohio, pointed out that the freedom of choice of a woman of color is relational and gender dynamic, and could be Christ-centered despite the atmosphere (Nygengele 2004, 28-71). For this to happen, first, the Christian woman recognized the various elements in culture, religion, and inherited tradition that oppressed her in her environment (Nygengele 2004, 30). Second, the woman comprehended her self-value and self-worth in God's love. This understanding brought inner healing and deliverance rather than striving for appreciation within a racially discriminating society (Nygengele 2004, 42-58). Finally, she handled the pain and suffering from career discrimination, dysfunctional family relations, and violent sociocultural conditions through her faith in God and affirmation from Bible-based pastors and pastoral caregivers (Nygengele 2004, 59).

Green stated that freedom of choice visually portrayed what controlled the woman's holistic choices: spirit, soul or body (Green 2008, 99). He noted the Apostle Paul's writing:

Indeed, the theme of Romans 6 is the inevitability of human slavery, with the only question being the identity of the master to whom one's life is presented: "to sin as instrument of wickedness" or "to God as instruments of righteousness" (v.13). As Paul reasons, "For just as you once presented your members as slaves to impurity and to greater and greater iniquity, so now present your members as slaves to righteousness for sanctification" (v. 19). Again: "Do you now know that if you present yourselves to anyone as obedient slaves, you are slaves of the one whom you obey, either of sin, which leads to death, or of obedience, which leads to righteousness?" (Green 2008, 99)

Therefore, the free choice of a woman of color in response to life's trials and tribulation need not be subsumed or suppressed by a corrupt judicial system, generational curses, or male supremacy (Green 2008, 102). Instead an African American woman's healthy lifestyle choices can be based upon her dependence on Jesus Christ, who provides her with stability in faith, reformation of self-identity in the Messiah, and the faith declaration of Scripture (Mitchem 2002, 113; Nyengele 2004, 201).

The theological perspective of an African American woman honoring and revering God through her healthy lifestyle reflects her Christ-like walk within her earthly relationships (Erickson 1998, 524). The healthcare maintenance of the woman of color before and after the slave trade period, was rooted upon her acceptance of her ancestors' holistic lifestyles integrating spirit, soul, and body (Tannenbaum 2012, 34; Gourdine 2011, 8-14). The influence from family tradition (during pre-and post-slave trades) and the effects of the healthcare deprivation, religious beliefs, lack of wellness knowledge, and modern medicine will be addressed in the historical section as it considered the impact of the antebellum period, the post-Civil War period, and the twentieth century.

Historical Foundation

Whenever you hear a story on the news about an unnecessary surgery or a mistake made on the operating table, a chill runs up your spine. This is true of anyone. All of us fear surgery; it's a human nature . . . For African Americans, this sort of public distrust is coupled with a more deeply imbedded personal trust, the origins of which span scores of prior generations. When hundreds of thousands of slaves arrive on these shore, an African woman's body was no longer her possession. It belonged to her master, and as such, its care was in his hands, not hers. If her temple was broken, beaten, and abused, if it was plagued by illness and disease, its trending was at her master's discretion. Melody T. McCloud, M.D., and Angela Ebron (McCloud and Ebron 2003, 5).

From generation to generation, women of African descent have relied upon their religious beliefs to overcome sickness and suffering from sinful practices (slavery) (Tannenbaum 2012, 33). During slavery, healthcare for African American women was dehumanizing and depressing (Tannenbaum 2012, 76). After the abolition of slavery, healthcare continued to be difficult for African American women to access. Transitioning into the twenty-first century, racial differences continue to influence the quality of life for African American women (Gourdine 2011, 8). This historical section will discuss how the Antebellum Era, the period from the American Civil War to 1890, and the events of the twentieth century (1890 on) impacted the lifestyles of African American women and their healthcare.

Antebellum Era: 1812-1861

Before the slave trade began, some women in African societies were treated as royalty and trail blazers (Patterson 2000,34). Before slave entrapment, the spiritual values of African women were rooted in their family religious beliefs, which often held that diseases, pain, and suffering resulted from sinful practices (Tannenbaum 2012, 33). Folk healing, the creative home-based medical healthcare, often dealt with superstitions, conjurations, and hoodoo practices (Patterson, 2000, 15; Tannenbaum 2012, 40).

Enslavement wrecked the woman of color's self-identity as she watched her health deteriorate (Mitchem 2007, 34; Patterson 2000, 39; Schwartz 2006, 31). Her body was not her own. Personal hygiene and medical care were based upon her master's decisions for slaves (Mitchem 2007, 52), and self-esteem was heavily impacted. Ultimately, slavery victimized the African woman's social, emotional, mental, spiritual and vocational wellbeing (Patterson 2000, 41; Ellison and Douglas 2010, 50).

Importing slaves ceased in 1808; however, southern states continued to utilize slave labor if the children were born in bondage (Schwartz 2006, 1). In slavery, women's bodies were degradingly labeled as grotesque. They were disrespected, used to fulfill their masters' sexual needs through rape, and forced into exploitation of labor by slave owners (Mitchem 2002, 13; Patterson 2000, 39-40; Volo and Volo 2004,19). Tannenbaum visually illustrated that the forced treatment of African American slaves was rooted in the masters' religion (Tannenbaum 2012, 31; Patterson 2000, 37). Within the slave society, African American women contributed to their masters' economic success through productive labor and procreation (Schwartz 2006,11). The women were not entitled to adequate medical services, since their masters did not value the relationship between religion and physical health (Tannenbaum 2012, 33).

This led to a lack of trust and confidence in their masters and hired physicians, as the women feared and resented their masters who forcibly controlled the most important feature of their physical life, their bodies (Schwartz 2006, 71; Lockley 2013, 648; Volo and Volo 2004, 18-19). The dominating white male leadership role caused the slave girl to live in isolation, to have feelings of low self-esteem, and to have a misunderstanding of God's healthy relationship plan between male and female (McConville 2016, 163-166; Patterson 2000,39; Volo and Volo 2004,18).

Since slave owners disrespected and mistreated African women's physical bodies, the women didn't trust the medical diagnoses of the physicians hired by the slave owners (Schwartz 2006, 71; Lockley 2013, 648). During this time, African American women's viewpoints of God's health plan for their physical bodies and intimate relationships between men and women were distorted (Volo and Volo 2004, 18). Medical coverage for African American women was provided only when beneficial to their slave owners, whose main purpose for offering the care of medical doctors was childbirth for plantation maintenance.

Because slave owners during the Antebellum time period did not have access to new supplies of slaves from Africa after 1808, they valued slave childbirth (Lockley 2013, 635). Medical doctors were used to oversee the health care of the enslaved women from puberty through the reproduction years for the followings purposes: to foster pregnancy, cure infertility, and resolve gynecological problems (Schwartz 2006, 67-290).

Breeding by force was acceptable to slave owners who wanted to improve the caretaking of their stock and increase their profits through the slave labor of men, women, and children (Byrd and Clayton 2000, 282). Medical care offered to female slaves was also used to identify and cure barrenness (Schwartz 2006, 30). During childbirth, white male doctors were there to ensure full term pregnancy and to treat complication from childbirth (Schwartz 2006, 28). The slave women received healthcare for the following diseases: tumors, cancer, and chronic or acute diseases (Schwartz 2006, 30). The personal hygiene of the African American woman was poor during this time, and she exhibited visual signs of inadequate nutrition before, during and after childbirth (Lockley 2013, 639). Due to maternal illness and the poor diet of infants throughout the weaning process, there was a high infant mortality rate (Lockley 2013, 640; Hill 2016, 32).

During the Antebellum era, the profits of the plantation owners were dependent upon slave labor. Barren slave women were labeled non-profitable, and barren women were resold, separated from loved ones, and beaten. They suffered emotionally, physically, and spiritually (Schwartz 2006, 93). For slaves who could bear children, repeated pregnancies introduced additional health issues such as miscarriage, abortions, and premature infants (Schwartz 2006, 108). The uncertainty of physicians regarding the moment when life begins for the infant led enslaved women to initiate fertility tests and herbal wisdom, which conflicted with the scientific knowledge of orthodox medical care practices by white physicians and threatened the ongoing expansion and profit within the southern society of the slave owners (Schwartz 2006, 110).

Multiple persons were needed during the birthing process. Midwives, female slaves, and slaveholders were involved in the labor areas (Long 2012, 12). Productivity depended upon successful childbirth among slaves; therefore, southern physicians were often required to be within the slave quarters during labor. In some cases, motherhood resulted in the female and newborn infant having health issues (Schwartz 2006, Long 2012, 21). Hemorrhaging resulted in the death of infants on arrival, and mothers experiencing extended labor. A quest for extensive health studies began, which led to the use of Caesarean sections (Schwartz 2006, 163). The health of the woman and infant were critically jeopardized when Caesarean sections were implemented (Schwartz 2006, 175). Her physical health, mental health, and general wellbeing were endangered from postnatal complications. Childbirth during the antebellum period often ended with the death of the mother or infant (Schwartz 2006,187; Long 2012, 22).

Civil War and Beyond (1861-1890)

The advent of the Civil War destroyed the institution of slavery (Ellison and Douglas 2010, 86). After years of bondage and dependency, the Emancipation Proclamation was issued on January 1, 1863, resulting in the African American woman being able to make her own choices in regards to her body and soul (Patterson 2000,41). Economic opportunities awakened much emotional and mental stress as the free woman faced the reality of limited career choice in the light of a lack of education and loss of housing (Ellison and Douglas 2010, 88). Post-Civil War, the African American woman's main employment status was categorized as "live in domestic servant" (Schwartz 2006, 290). Within this environment, living conditions reverted to the former environment prevalent during the days of slavery. Life for the African American woman continued to mean sexual exploitation, poor health care and medical coverage, poverty, and low self-esteem (Schwartz 2006, 291).

Mistrust of health care professionals among African American families originated during slavery and continued during and after the Civil War. African American women publicly expressed their fears about their bodies being used for research testing. They found it hard to believe in the authenticity of assigned physicians (McCloud and Ebron 2003,5; Dr. Golubic 2016, Interview).

These women had hoped that deliverance from their masters' dehumanizing treatment and control over their lifestyle would come when the institution of slavocracy ended (Ellison and Douglas 2010, 86; Thompson 1987, 131).

> When the war finally broke out, it brought with it, on one hand advances in surgery and emancipation of thousands of slaves. Simultaneously, these African Americans were thrust into living conditions in southern cities and in Union army and contraband camps that would make good health nearly impossible. Alongside these medical developments, however, the cultural connections between medicine and dependency persisted. Slaves themselves, once free, quickly found that white doctors and public health officials, like white masters and the doctors they had employed, demanded compliance with their medical regimes and held African American traditional herbal healing in low regard. Issues of control and autonomy remained paramount as African Americans struggled to define themselves as free people within medical culture (Long 2012, 43).

In the post-Civil War era, African American women feared that past medical experiments and exploitations would resurface. The African American women remembered the Antebellum medical experiments where their ancestors were used to find remedies for sun-stroke, blister cure, and eye diseases. These tests left African Americans with severe body burns, uncontrollable bleeding, and loss of eyesight and limps (Hogue, Hargraves, and Collins 2000, 13). The health disparity from the Jim Crow laws meant the continued neglect of African American's health care concerns, self-worth, and self-value (Thompson 1987, 265). The dehumanizing medical treatments and laws caused African American women to doubt the Caucasian medical doctors' health diagnosis, medical prescriptions, and physicians' referrals (White 2011, 212; Washington 2008, 54).

In the early years after the Civil War, freedom from the slave trade did not necessarily improve conditions, and resulted in sicknesses, diseases, and prolonged starvation for approximately 500,000 freed slaves (Downs 2012, 23). African Americans who transitioned from slavery to freedom experienced physical, mental, emotional, and spiritual stress. They feared the unknown, the effects of healthcare based on medical practice, federal government policy, and competition in the labor force (Downs 2012, 43).

Epidemic diseases ran rampant within the African American communities. Soldiers were vulnerable to scabies, skin conditions, and overwhelming physical and emotional stress since their living conditions provided inadequate sanitation and hygiene (Tannenbaum 2012, 177; Long 2012, 45). The federal government had insufficient healthcare, medical coverage, and medicinal facilities for freed African American soldiers and their families (Downs 2012, 36; Tannenbaum 2012, 188; Long 2012, 48). The war's effects left unhealthy marks on African American families that included physical harm, germ warfare, malnourishment, mental issues, vocational stress, lack of education, emotional harm, and fear of returning to slave entrapment (Long 2012, 55; Tannenbaum 2012, 197).

Despite the racial inequalities within the subsequent Jim Crow era, the newly freed African American women survived by working as nurses, laundresses, cooks, and maintenance keepers on farms and plantations (Forbes 1998, 51). Due to lack of education and career skills, African American women faced numerous occupational hazards. Some were forced to work as prostitutes, and occupational prostitution created the need for healthcare to address the spread of venereal disease. Industrial manufacturing jobs exhausted the women's physical strength without therapeutic coverage (Tannenbaum 2012, 111; Ellison and Douglas 2010, 89).

Although the war had been meant to change conditions for the former slaves, the career opportunities and healthcare appeared to be little different from the Antebellum era. In 1865, the War Department created the Freedmen's Bureau which was meant to help freed slaves work through the challenges of emancipation: social, economic, educational, political, and medical (Downs 2012, 45). However, the federal government still denied responsibility for the medical care of freed slaves. Consequently, African Americans returned to their ancestors' folk healing remedies to deal with issues of wellness, healing, racism, daily challenges, and spiritual support (Mitchem 2007, 164). Black folk healing helped the woman of African descent to endure the white man's treatment and taught her how to harmonize relationships within her new season (Mitchem 2007, 167; 71).

Freedom hospitals provided freed slaves and African American veterans with temporary care such as shelter, food, clothing and primitive medical treatment. The federal government's subsequent decision to limit aid led to over-populated hospitals, unpaid medical fees, and slaves working in a free labor environment (Downs 20102, 87; Tannenbaum 2012, 189). The prison-like almshouse, an extension of freedom hospitals, became the free slaves' place of refuge when they were desperate and did not have a family support system (Tannenbaum 20102,195). Receiving medical care seemed impossible since free people's income could not cover the fees of the doctors who worked for the bureau. To assist them, the physicians of the bureau collaborated and converted the hospitals' outer perimeter of land plots into vegetable gardens that provided nourishment for their patients and free slaves, while providing them employment as sales persons (Downs 2012,89; Long 2012, 148-149).

The Western Sanitary Commission, the North-Western Freedmen's Aid, and the Colored Benevolent Societies worked together during the emancipation to help freed people overcome the destructive living conditions of slavery (Long 2012, 100; Downs 2012, 90). These charitable organizations helped the African American population to develop and adapt a health and wellness plan within their daily activities (Tannenbaum 2012, 199; Forbes 1998, 113). They provided African Americans with health coverage, shelter, and employment (Forbes 1998, 52; Downs 2012, 87).

Disappointment in limited medical coverage given to free people led the African American women to develop entrepreneurial skills in organizing and networking. This led to professional and institutional healthcare for African Americans provided by African American women (Forbes 1998, 67; Long 2012, 139). As active healthcare providers, these free women dedicated their time and talents to educating newly freed slaves on the topic of self-preservation. This helped to eliminate the fears and dangers of falling into poverty (Downs 2012, 65; Mitchem 2007, 47).

The African American elite society implemented various benevolence organizations to support the Colored Orphan Asylum and Association, poverty stricken free slaves, payment of unpaid medical expenses, and educational institutions. They established goodwill organizations which dealt with healthcare and poverty among the recently freed people (Forbes 1998, 77). The medical industry during the Civil War period did not shelter or comfort the African American women from the enormous suffering experienced from the war's medical crisis, discriminative labor laws, and smallpox epidemic (Downs 2012,112; Long 2012, 66). Despite the continuing challenges, the development of a holistic lifestyle for the African American woman became more promising as she transitioned into the twentieth century.

Twentieth Century (1890-present)

After the Jim Crow period, access to American health care continued to be influenced by skin color, affecting the patients' medical treatment, services, and life span. The prominence of lynching, as well as mass killings such as the Slocum Massacre, shortened the lifespan of African Americans. In 1901 in east Texas, between eight to twenty-two African American were lynched, the Slocum Massacre (Bills 2014, 12-26). The racial barriers within the social, economic, and political realms resulted in mental health disparities among the people of color (Lowe 2006, 29).

While the federal government in the state of Texas showed disinterest in public safety for freed African Americans, the healthcare neglect resulted in continuous misdiagnosis, restricted medical services, and unethical and exploitive clinical research projects such as the Tuskegee experiment (Bills 2014, 80-81; Anekwe 2015, 621). The Tuskegee experiment was conducted from 1932 to 1972. It studied the effects of untreated syphilis on impoverished, rural, African-American males (Downs 2012, 159).

> Of the various racial and ethnic minorities, though, African Americans were, for various reasons, by far the most thoroughly scrutinized. Given the long history in America of racial prejudice, it wasn't a surprise that blacks were especially subject to inferior treatment. Compared with whites, they had lower rates of cardiac surgeries, fewer hip and knee replacements, fewer kidney and liver transplants. Diabetic blacks were more often amputated than diabetic whites. Non-diabetic blacks were amputated more often too. Blacks were more likely to receive open surgeries rather than the less dangerous laparoscopic procedures. (White 2011, 212)

African American medical schools and primary care physicians were scarce (Byrd and, Clayton 2001, 215). Yet the racial killings and the lack of preventive medical and dental coverages did not stop African American women from pursuing vocation, education, and self-preservation within a dominant white society (Mitchem 2004, 121).

The determination and endurance of African American women was seen in their willingness to seek knowledge about wellness, holistic care, and medical cures, and to get over cultural differences within the dominant white society which determined healthcare within society's medical institutions.

> Something occurs in addition to the medication, cause I don't think that medication heals. I think that's just one small piece of helping us move on that continuum, but the healing aspect is greater. So, when I see repeaters, there's no healing there. Even when symptoms re-occur, the people that have had some healing experience it differently… They've got tumors, but they've been healed. They feel they are at a point where healing has occurred. They die peaceful. It's a different level I think in terms of healing. We don't begin to really touch that a lot in health, in Western medicine. (Mitchem 2004, 120).

The concern of African American women for the healthcare of their families and communities led them to become medical trainers, to bring racial uplift (Shakir 2016, Lecture). History-making African American women doctors, such as Rebecca Crumple and Rebecca Cole, graduated from New England Medical Female College, and were advocates who promoted social activism through freed women collaboration (Shakir, 2016, Lecture; Mitchem 2004, 127).

The professional African American women voluntarily offered educational courses on health and wellness in the areas of hygiene, physical health care, nutrition, and mental, and emotional healings. The purpose for the ongoing continuing education courses for African American women as medical trainers was to motivate them through their struggles with and within a dominant white society. This helped the African American women to maintain their cultural heritage and self-identity in Christ (Mitchem 2004, 129; Johnson 1998, 111). Freed women who survived the slave trade period also realized that within a masculine society they ranked the lowest in terms of social status and occupational standing (Haggard 2010, 41).

The false self-identity portrayed through racism and healthcare transitioned from the slave entrapment period, through the Antebellum era, through the Civil War. Its aftermath continued into the twentieth century and affected the freed woman's holistic lifestyle (Haggard 1998, 149). Yet the true identity of an African American woman was revealed through her sacrificial health and wellness lifestyle.

Other factors were at play as well. The social structures of African American women were impacted as their living conditions transitioned from a rural to urban environment. This affected nutrition habits, sleeping accommodations, the job market, religious rituals, and family intimacies (Mitchem 2007, 55). Women who were accustomed to eating meals that were leftovers from the master's table, now had to purchase food. African American women also had to transition from forced labor to unemployment. Their lack of financial income resulted in living in congested environments, sharing unsanitary restrooms, and receiving health care from Caucasian physicians who were racist (Byrd and Clayton 2000, 351). The women may have been freed from the mental and physical abuse of slavery; yet they were now faced with survival, personal provision, and healthcare necessities for themselves and their families. Meal planning, seeking employment, the needs for transportation, and medical coverage were now part of daily life (Mitchem 2007, 58).

Health and wellness proclamation statements were used throughout the community to help their culture to develop and maintain healthier living conditions (Johnson1998,1-33). Freedom's Journal, the first African American owned and operated newspaper, was used to bring unity between African American leaders and their communities, and to allow African-American voices to be heard on a variety of topics (Haggard 2010, 189).

The literary voices of African American women recreated their ancestors' medical coverages, health plans, and historical events that the white culture neglected and failed to recognize (Hull, Scott and Smith 1982, 190, 208-260). As examples of these voices, psychologist and author Dr. Brenda Wade revealed how black women learned and dealt with "depression through displaced anger," resentment from racism, sexism and classism (Hoytt and Beard 2012, 146). Medical doctor Melody T. McCloud educated African American women on the "top five medical concerns" they may endure due to stressful relationships or situations, unhealthy living, and genetic transference (McCloud 2010,19).

In the late twentieth century, the United States worked to eliminate the racial barrier within the health care system by passing the Civil Rights Act (1964) and amending Social Security (1965) with Medicare-Medicaid coverage (Thompson 2015, 278). Advocates Dula and Goering proclaimed that the unifying cry of the African American woman is "It just ain't fair" in relation to their treatment within the American health care system (Dula and Goering 1994, 7). The United States government offered minimal incentives to private medical practitioners who presented medical services to the disenfranchised African American women (Dula and Goering 1994, 125). Affordable health care for minorities did not eliminate health disparities between the African American and Causation populations (Hogue, Hargraves, and Collins 2000 102).

From slave entrapment through the twentieth century, the "whole person" plan for African American women incorporated holistic strategies. African American educators offered lessons for freed people centered around acceptance of self-worth, self-respect, identity, dignity in spite of racism, income suppression, discrimination from politicians, and medical plans and labor laws (Johnson, Pitre, and Johnson 2014, 123). Ongoing spiritual cleansing, accepting contentment in suffering, receiving healing through forgiveness, and overcoming evil were necessities that needed to be addressed (Hull, Scott, and Smith 1982, 103, 115, 141).

Summary

This chapter discussed the biblical, theological, and historical foundations for this project in relation to the African Americans woman's holistic lifestyle. Daily survival for African American women was rooted in their spiritual belief in God's eord (Koptak 2003, 680; 3 John 1:2), utilizing passages such as Proverbs 31 and the letters of Paul. The theological perspective considered the importance of purpose, anthropological views, and the concept of freedom of choice. The historical section explored how the healthcare needs of the freed people became their responsibility and included more than just physical fitness, nutrition, and self-medication. The next chapter, the relevant contemporary works, will examine the components of holistic living within the lifestyles of African American women.

CHAPTER THREE

REVIEW OF THE LITERATURE

Women of God can never be like women of the world. The world has enough
women who are tough; we need women who are tender. There are enough
women who are coarse; we need women who are kind. There are enough
women who are rude; we need women who are refined. We have enough
women of fame and fortune; we need more women of faith.
We have enough greed; we need more goodness. We have enough vanity;
we need more virtue. We have enough popularity; we need more purity. (*A
Woman of* God, quoted by Margaret D. Nadauld, in *The Joy of Womanhood*,
2015)

Who is the African American woman in the twenty-first century? Is she to be,
as Margaret Nadauld suggests, (*from* the quote above, *A Woman of God*) a tender,
kind, refined woman of faith? Should she be, as I would suggest, a complete woman
who values her self-worth, and celebrates and cheers other women on their journey
toward self-acceptance? As a person who is a spirit, has a soul, and lives within a
physical body, what impact do these three components have on our identity in
Christ? Consequently, the ongoing question for African American women, especially
related to their health care, is this: how they can continue to represent the Messiah
in spirit, soul, and body?

The answer is found within the purpose of this project, to impact the
healthcare of women within the Union-Miles community in Cleveland, Ohio by
providing six weeks of holistic workshops that help participants integrate God's
Divine Wellness Plan into their daily lives. The contemporary foundations section will
illustrate how experts in the fields of the spirit, soul and body suggest that African
American women, living within a fast-paced society, within the natural world, can
maintain their faith walk. The following dimensions of wellness will be addressed
within the three components of holistic lifestyle: spirit (relationship with God), soul
(mind frame and emotional state), and body (healthcare and self-care).

Spirit

How can an African American woman of faith survive and thrive within
contemporary society? Patricia Gundry says that a female Christian lifestyle requires
a woman to spiritually mimic her Messiah at home, within her career, and by herself
(Gundry 1981, 228). Richard Foster suggests that her support system is rooted
within her ongoing personal relationship with God. Foster comments that her own
self-acceptance of who she is in Christ motivates her to develop and maintain a

spiritual connection with the Son of Man, Jesus Christ. Spending time with God helps her to grow through her daily process of spiritual transformation. This conversion is progressive and possible as she encounters God through meditation on the Bible and engagement in the self-awakening process (Foster 2008, 44). A focus on spiritual development will include an intentional engagement in the self-awakening process, regular study and interaction with scripture, and a commitment to prayer.

Self-Development in Christ

According to David Benner, the true identity of all people depends upon their stages of self-development in Christ (Benner 2012, 156). Richard Foster concurs that a woman's holistic journey in relation to the awakening self will be contingent upon her attentiveness and acceptance of God's presence through the Holy Spirit's guidance (Foster 2008, 85). Eugene Peterson says that knowing the voice of God is an essential component needed for a woman to make decisions that lead to self-preservation in the areas of socialization, vocation, and ministry. Peterson adds that the women's lifestyle choices depend upon their knowledge, acceptance, and commitment to abide by God's wellness blueprint (Peterson 2006, 23).

According to Gregory Boyd, a person's choice to walk, serve, and live for Christ revolves around living in the present moment. Her wellness and survival rests upon her ability to accept her self-image, given to her through God's grace which is found within the Scriptures. Regarding spiritual nutrition, Boyd notes that a believer who mimics Christ throughout her physical activities reveals God's Kingdom in the present moment. First, the saint's daily interactions, breaths, and movements are impossible without God's presence. Second, God is the God of the living and not the "God of the already past or the God of the not-yet-present" (Boyd 2010, 18). Finally, the Christian woman's health choices become a "living sacrament" through her submission to God's divine wellness plan. As a result, she experiences her Messiah's love, joy, and peace (Boyd 2010, 18). Boyd defines how to communicate with God; however, his information does not reveal how to make daily application of one's biblical knowledge (spiritual insight), to one's health choices concerning both body and soul (Boyd 2010, 18).

Jay Adams explains that true self-identity is grounded within God's word. Before women can help others on their spiritual journey, their lifestyles must incorporate a healthy biblically-based understanding of self-image, self-esteem, and self-love. He indicates that a woman seeking God's heart authentically develops and maintains her self-worth and self-value, which is accomplished through self-denial of the flesh and acceptance of God's mercy and grace. This Christlike self-image is formed as the woman walks in a spirit of humility, maintaining sober mindedness, a

44

non-judgmental attitude, and respect for others. He says that the self-esteem and self-love of women can be rooted in their belief system. Adam indicates that this self-esteem and self-love enables them to proclaim that their healthy choices are made through the righteousness of Christ (Adams 1986, 118).

In summary, Benner, Foster, Peterson, and Adam concur that self-development in Christ manifests within belief values and practices. They agree that a woman's healthy self-image revolves around her biblically-based understanding of self-image, self-worth, and self-esteem in Christ. They collectively express that its intentional choices, the self-image can be formed around the scriptures.

Scripture

Adams also suggests that a daily dose of scripture reassured believers that their true-self-identity was not based on preconceived self-worth, self-pride, or self-work (Adams 1986, 118). Tarry Wardle adds that the woman's intimate relationship with God makes a difference in how she handles spiritual matters within a real society and how her lifestyle reveals the scriptures. He says that daily scripture readings impact self-perception which can guard from a self-centered lifestyle. Wardle teaches how self-centeredness (small ego self) is a strategic way to manipulate and control one's freedom of choices Wardle's emphasis is that throughout the Scriptures, God's love is the core. This becomes a central theme for holistic living (Wardle, 2016, 26). Howard Thurman says that loving oneself from a biblical perspective brings redemption from generational curses, a gift especially to African American women who live under the curse not only of their own family history, but also of the curses brought through slavery. Thurman states that historically, God's love has helped African American women to endure spiritual, emotional, and physical suppression. It offered reassurance during slavery, employment discrimination, and sexual abuse (Thurman 1976, 84).

Stephanie Mitchem notes that Christian hope sustained African American women as they were being dehumanized and oppressed within the healthcare system and in labor force (Mitchem 2004, 26). Also, womanist theologian Renita Weems explained how African American women have related their life experiences to the various female Bible characters. Weems proclaims that African American women have related to Hagar's story of "exploitation and persecution" (Weems 1988, 1). She adds that the cry of shame experienced by Jephthah is reality for every woman who embraced deception through a loved one's ambition for power and prestige. Weems demonstrates that Jesus offered a healing touch to women who suffered from poor health or bad reputations. Jesus' healing touch included the adulterous woman, "woman with the interminable menstrual flow, and women with five husbands" (Weems 1988, 93). Daniel Simundson agrees that the personal lifestyles of female biblical characters encouraged and motivated African American women to continue their belief and faith walk in Christ regardless of their health challenges, sexual mistreatments, and family issues (Simundson 1982, 333).

Boyd states that African American women maintained balanced lifestyles when they acknowledged that their self-images belonged to them as gracious gifts from God (Boyd 2010, 149). African American women whose lifestyle incorporated healthy Bible-based interpretation of their self-image, self-esteem, and self-love were then able to motivate and encourage other women on their spiritual journeys. These women proclaimed that their holistic choices made through the righteousness of Christ were manifested because of what were their daily selective choices to meditate on God's word. Thurman expresses that Jesus (the Scripture in flesh) was a member of the minority group; therefore, the African American women's receptiveness of Jesus' presence and His love for them helped them to deal with racism and discrimination against them as a minority group. God's *agape* love for them enabled them to endure spiritual, emotional, and physical suppressions (Thurman 1996, 8).

Adams and Wardle agree that a daily dose of Scripture encourages and reminds God's children that regardless of their life challenges, their true identity and shelter is in Him. The contribution of Weems and Mitchem to the discussion of the importance of ongoing Scripture reading is that African American women could relate to the various life challenges that female biblical characters experienced. Finally, Thurman expresses that Jesus' experiences with rejection and physical suppression during His earthly ministry brought comfort and encouragement to a minority group who were enduring spiritual, emotional, and physical destruction. This discussion of spirit indicates that the minority group can find comfort, strength and reassurance within the scripture.

Prayer

A holistic lifestyle for African American women also revolves around their effectual, fervent, Bible-based prayers. Contemporary life can challenge daily decisions, both personally and professionally in areas such as time management, unknown financial needs, health issues, and family conflicts. Catherine Musgrave, Carol Allen, and Gregory Allen state that in the search for answers to their daily life challenges, African American women have historically sought God's guidance through prayer and continue to do so in today's world, as they "hold belief in God and prayer to be health-protective behaviors" (Musgrave, Allen and Allen 2002, 558). When African American women have conversations with God, they find comfort in their times of grief, they overcome feelings of anger, and they release hurts from abusive relationships. This intimate chat with God allows the African American woman to find her identity, since her personal struggles for self-identity can be an ongoing battle (Musgrave, Allen and Allen 2002, 557).

As African American women ask themselves about self-knowledge and identity, they can do so in prayer. The words of the song, *I Know Who I Am* are an example of the result of a prayer of faith.

> We are a chosen generation. We've been called forth to show His excellence. All I require for life, God has given me and I know who I am. I know who God says I am. What He says I am. Where He says I'm at. I know who I am. I'm walking in power. I'm working miracles. I live a life of favor, for I know I am. Oh oh oh, oh oh I know who I am. I am righteous oh…. I am so rich, I am beautiful. I'm walking in power. I'm working miracles. I live a life of favor, for I know who I am. Take a look at me. I'm a wonder. It doesn't matter what you see now. Can you see His glory? For I know who I Am. (Sinach, 2012)

African American women continuously seek godly counsel through prayer. They seek self-knowledge and the solutions for life's struggles. That is why prayer through singing is often helpful and appropriate. Advocate Grace Cornish says that as the African American woman is appealing to her Messiah, this helps her to look at herself through the spiritual and physical mirror without judgement. Throughout the generations, African American women have lifted their hands and heart to heaven and prayed vociferously for help in maintaining peaceful minds while they endured racism, discrimination, and family separation, and continue to do so in the twenty-first century (Cornish 2002, 191).

Cornish suggests that an African American woman can find love, respect, and self-worth through communication with God. Cornish believes that prayer has helped herself and other African American women overcome societal pressures, past abusive relationships, and suppression within the career world due to male chauvinism. Cornish's prayer slogan is "praying power guarantees staying power" (Cornish 2002, 193).

As African American women added ongoing Bible-based prayer requests to their daily lifestyles, they realized that their contemporary lifestyles were challenging when making decisions within their personal and professional lifestyles. Norvella Carter and Matthew Parker recognize that the Bible-based prayer requests reinforced the ability of the African American women to listen and respond to God's guidance in making good choices that involved such things as time management, financial distributions, health issues, family decisions, and self-identity (Carter and Parker 1996, 245). Prayer was a key factor that aided the African American women on the various Christ-like ways to interact within their society, and they concur that the women struggled emotionally from being victims of racism, classism, and sexism, yet they dealt with mood swings by engaging in spiritual checkup and soul-searching (Carter and Parker 1996, 245). Mitzi Smith adds that African American women were able to overcome past mental, emotional, and physical abuse suffered through racism and sexism when they spent time with God, walked in His Sprit, and remembered His grace and love (Smith 2015, 160).

Carter and Parker add that the African American woman who prays is able to accept her self-worth, as she displays visual integrity and genuine love when servng others (Carter and Parker 1996,54). Eleanor Hoytt and Hilary Beard state that the African American Christian women realize their health and wellbeing are secure in God's life-giving words (Hoytt and Beard 2012, 314). Also, Dallas Willard concurs that declaring the Scriptures through prayer was the antidote used for the renovation of the woman's heart when engaging in soul-searching (Willard 2012, 30).

To summarize, the authors conclude their discussion on the necessity of a fervent prayer lifestyle for the African American women in agreement that prayer was used as a survival tool. Musgrave, Allen and Allen stated that the African American women's prayer communication with God was used to maintain their spiritual health and daily survival. Cornish confirm that The African American women comfort during their daily life struggles came through songs of prayer. Carter and Parker and Hoytt and Beard express how the African American women found their self-worth, health and wellbeing through their Bible-based prayers. Willard concludes that prayer was the spiritual antidote used by many to endure life struggles, soul comfort, and cleansing.

Soul

Carter and Parker reference how African American women, past and present, have been victims of racism, classism, and sexism which have negatively impacted their emotional and mental well-being. The ongoing practice of 'isms' violated their spiritual belief, resulting in colorism attacks, and even extend to such practical areas as self-disapproval of their hair length and texture. They discuss how the ism labels often resulted in an attack on the African American woman's self-worth, intellectual ability, and emotional state, the soul. Since self-care of the soul is essential for inner healthcare maintenance, the following topics will be discussed in regard to the soul, mind and emotion: the recognition of thought processes, understanding of the role of racism and sexism, and the relief of stress (Carter and Parker 1996, 245).

Recognition of Thought Process

Wardle's seminary lecture called *Identity Integrity and the Awakening of the True Self* explained how destructive thoughts that are permitted to linger result in emotional turmoil, leading to a false conception of self. Wardle spoke about the result of fear and anxiety ending in an emotional imbalance; however, thoughts can be controlled by the renewing of the mind through God's Word (Wardle 2001, 179). Willard adds that by engaging in regular reading of scripture a person who is dealing with emotional imbalance can begin a journey of self-recovery within his or her mind (Willard 2012, 96).

Angela Neal-Barnett points out that the destructive thought process that comes from asking the question, "What if?" causes anxiety, suggesting the unhealthy lifestyle associated with ongoing worrying about the unknown becomes as natural as breathing. Throughout generations, African-American women who have engaged in the "what if" syndrome have obsessed over the following concerns: past failures being exposed, job discrimination, provisions for their families, marital relationships, and housing. Neal-Barnett began to offer psychology courses to educate African American women on how to overcome negative thoughts, the fear of failures, financial difficulties, and family challenges (Neal-Barnett 2003, 50-66).

Neal-Barnett's psychological approach for a healthy mind incorporated several steps. First, a volunteer health survey was offered. The survey included a self and family history in the following areas: depression, anxiety, behavior patterns, and medication. A second step included spiritual meditation and music therapy. Third was a negative thought tracking monitor accomplished through journaling. Fourth, ongoing prayer for the purpose of overcoming negative patterns was taught. Finally, transitioning from depression, anxiety, or feelings of failure to healthy constructive thoughts was addressed (Neal-Barnett 2003, 147).
She adds that healthy constructive thoughts became possible when the African American women were able to renew their minds daily through these components, as well as spending time in God's word and walking in His Spirit (Neal-Barnett 2003, 147).

Wardle and Neal-Barnett agree that the "what if" syndrome and destructive thoughts result in emotional stress and false conception of self-identity. They both agree that deliverance from negative thinking, racism and sexism is possible for African American women through the renewing of their minds through Scripture and knowing that Jesus is walking with them.

Role of Racism and Sexism

Mitzi Smith discusses how African American women often face stereotypes and images that are an obvious or subtle result of a combination of racism and sexism (Smith 2015, 160). As an example, obstetrician and gynecologist Melody McCloud found that national and international media images of African American women are negative and stereotypical. According to McCloud, traditionally colorism visually displayed favoritism towards lighter complexion African American women, as women of lighter complexions were favored as newscasters, as dating preference for African American men, and as movie actors (McCloud 2010, 244). Carter and Parker add that the physical appearance of women was not respected or accepted within their personal or professional circle (Carter and Parker 1996, 59).

Smith and McCloud concur that the role of racism and sexism promoted colorism which favored light complexion African American women. Both Thurman and Villarosa agree that dependency on the Messiah's presence helped the African American woman to deal with the prejudicial stereotypes, healthcare restrictions, and racist job market. Thurman encouraged African-American women to have reverent fear of Christ, suggesting that their relationship with the Messiah would help them to overcome the many types of fears of deception and oppression within their environment, and the prejudicial stereotypes that continued to make life more difficult for African American women (Thurman 1976, 26).

As Thurman understood, the fear of slave entrapment, an abusive medical system, a racist job market, and unsanitary living conditions spanned generation from slavery into the present. The fear of physical violence towards African American women caused negative emotions, which restricted the possibility of having successful and healthy lifestyles (Thurman 1976, 30). Linda Villarosa notes as well that the heavy responsibility of being a strong African American woman often was understood as requiring her to surrender her wellbeing, emotional health, physical fitness, and spiritual growth (Villarosa 1994, 367).

Villarosa adds that taking on the role as a caretaker, African American women gave priority to the healthcare concerns of others before themselves: spouses, children, parents, lovers, and elders. This health care prioritization resulted in African American women suffering with emotional agony in the areas of severe depression, stress, and anxiety (Villarosa 1994, 371). Both Villarosa and Bell Hooks note that the ongoing emotional wellbeing of African American women has been affected by society's message of self-hate toward them (Hooks 2015, 12; Villarosa 1994, 370).

Hooks recognizes that relationship break-ups also played a part in the false self-identity in African American women. This identity crisis meant that the woman's self-image was based upon the opinion of family members and society's acceptance or rejection of their self-identity. This is seen in the areas of physical appearance, financial status, and educational achievements (Hooks 2015, 19). Both Hooks and Villarosa realize that for the African American woman, boldness to stand up for herself was suppressed through abuse, punishment, and loss of control over her physical body through white supremacy (Hooks 2015, 20; Villarosa 1994, 369).

Hooks, Johnson, Hogue, Hargraves, and Collins comment on how unhealthy medical coverage were generational. They all concur that the role of racism and sexism resulted with the African American women suffering from emotional agony, anxiety and in need of stress relief. Yet African American women were able to engage in health care maintenance when they researched and learned their families' medical histories. Yvonne Johnson, Carol Hogue, Martha Hargraves, and Karen Scott Collins discuss how chronic diseases, unhealthy eating habits, and lifestyle rituals transitioned from generation to generation; yet as the African American women became aware of their families' unhealthy lifestyles and medical issues through offered educational healthcare information, which helped them to be responsible for their own well-being (Johnson 1998, 142; Hogue, Hargraves, and Collins 2000, 246).

Stress Relief

As can be seen from the challenges facing African American women, the role of stress needed to be recognized. Medical physician Helen Derosis advised African American women to routinely engage in a holistic stress-reduction strategy. This approach eliminated the pressure from tension and exposed the situations or fear that triggered the attack (Derosis 1998, 32). Villarosa and Derosis offer the following holistic steps for stress relief: identifying a troublesome issue, seeking God for a solution, obeying the Holy Spirit's intervention, engaging in mediation for calmness, pampering of the self, and being a part of a Christian support group. These self-help techniques encouraged African American women to heal their wounds spiritual, physically and emotionally through their faith in God's word and behavioral changes they were encouraged to institute (Villarosa 1994, 372; Derosis 1998, 68).

Villarosa states that over the centuries, stress release for African American women has come through music, beginning with the spiritual comfort and communication through religious songs during the years of slavery (Villarosa 1994, 398). Bell Hooks adds that for many generations, African American women were taught that full exposure of their emotions endangered their survival within a white man's society and had the belief that showing fear within their community illustrated their selfish needs (Hooks 2015, 101). Yet music allowed for a release of those emotions. According to Ruth Feldstein, during the Civil Rights movement, Lena Horne fought black oppression through her singing and acting career which emphasized her politicization and activism on behalf of civil rights between 1963 and 1965 (Feldstein 2013, 11).

In this decade, Beverly Bond, former model turned DJ, is using her non-profit organization called Black Girls Rock to build the self-esteem of young African American women through music, mentoring, and art projects (Bond 2006, Breakthrough Women). In 2016, singer, songwriter, and actress Beyoncé Giselle Knowles-Carter illustrated her insight on the physical and mental abuse of African American women within society through her music videos. The film version of

51

Lemonade revealed Beyoncé's expression of southern African American women's lifestyle as they transitioned through the rural and urban south from the period of the slave trade through the Antebellum period, and into the twentieth and then twenty-first century, allowing her to speak up for African American women today (Knowles 2016, video).

To summarize, African Americans tried to maintain wellbeing within their spirit and mind through religious songs, musical entertainment, and stress relief techniques. Derosis and Villarosa offer the African American women healing through holistic stress relief steps. Contemporary artists such as Beverly Bond and Beyoncé Giselle Knowles-Carter offer support through mentorship, videos, and art projects that educate African American women in the awareness of mental and health abuse. Yet, the unique healing power of holiness, soul cleansing, and self-acceptance for the African American women did not always extend to their physical appearance. For a healing of spirit, soul and body, the God within and His approval of the African American women's bodies must be graciously revealed and accepted by the African American women. This will be outlined in the next section.

Body

Black women's relationship to our bodies is complex and often vexed. We take a lot of trouble to look good, yet we don't always do the things that will keep our bodies toned and strong. We have a healthier concept of weight overall than women of other races -- in that we don't subscribe to the ideal of thin-is-beautiful -- yet we're more likely to be overweight than any other group, and we are disproportionately affected by weight-related diseases such as diabetes and hypertension. We have rich cultural tradition around food, yet we often eat the wrong things for the wrong reasons, and social and economic facts make it hard for us to feed ourselves and our families well, even when we want to. We lead lives that keep us running, yet few of us get the exercise we should. We're more likely than women of other races to say we feel good about ourselves no matter what -- yet like, Dr. Downer's [Dr. Goulda Downer] audience, we turn away from our reflection in the mirror. (Hoytt and Beard 2012, 247)

Through their encounters with racism, slave entrapment, and discrimination, African American women often received poor medical care. Melody McCloud and Angele Ebron report that African American women were of higher risk for chronic disease, in part because of a lack of education in health care coverages (McCloud and Ebron 2003, 2). They agree that health care through self-care is an ongoing challenge for African American women. The lack information, education, and income limited the women's medical access to general physicians, health-care providers, conventional medicine, alternative healing care, life insurance and burial policies, and saving investment plans (Hoytt and Beard 2012, 331). Smith adds that slavery and post-slavery America left the African American women demeaned (Smith 2015, 164). Evelyn White remarks that physical abuse caused the African American women to feel disrespected. Sexual abuse brought on embarrassment, shame, and lack of self-confidence, as they were not in control of their own bodies (White 1985, 11). For African American women to practice self-care so that they could achieve well-being in their bodies, they needed to educate themselves to understand such things as health risk factors and the health care operational system.

Health Care

Mitchem states that the health history of African American women is impacted by their families and communities. The negative effects of the American health care system within the African American culture has been publicly exposed through the AIDS crisis, the lack of minority health care providers, unaffordable medical coverages, and limited knowledge on the social differences between African and White Americans (Mitchem 2004, 133).

Hogue, Hargraves and Collins express that the mission of the health care industry is to offer preventative care, cure disease, and educate African American women about various health risk factor, such as diabetes, heart disease, kidney disease, obesity, stroke and physical violence. These negative health conditions have led African American women to have higher rates of mortality, stress, disability, shame, and lack of self-confidence (Hogue, Hargraves, and Collins 2000, 234).

Contemporary health care for African American women often required them to seek medical care from Caucasian physicians. In many instances, the Caucasian medical doctors stereotyped the health needs of African American women based on their perception of African American culture, and the individual medical needs of the women were not recognized, a situation that Augustus White, an orthopedic surgeon, labeled "divesting, shocking, and a form of inequality" (White 2011, 211). In one attempt to address this issue, White states that health disparity committees were formed to serve as liaisons to bring equality of health care through two new directives: Directive 21 and Directive 22. The directives educated and addressed the bias of physicians and trainees in their understanding about the healthcare needs of African American women (White 2011, 258-259). Shirley Hill adds that African American women are currently trying to overcome doctor and patient trust issues (Hill 2016, 89).

Hogue, Hargraves and Collins state that the health care reform act sought to provide a competitive medical coverage market for African American and Hispanic women. They express that the bill dealt with the racial disparities in women's health coverage. It offered access to benefits of health and dental coverage through employment and implemented fair eligibility standards which ensured that African American women receive necessary health coverage. Yet, health care providers for women of African descent are still not as available as they are for Caucasian women (Hogue, Hargraves and Collins 2000, 97-112).

Naomi Johnson says that African American health supporters are educating African American women on how to take responsibility for their own. Yet even though each day on earth reminds African American women that their physical bodies should represent Christ, they still are struggling with maintaining self-care (Johnson 2013, 142).

Natasha Tarpley suggests that an African American woman's self-acceptance starts with looking in the mirror and realizing that a holistic lifestyle is an ongoing process (Tarpley 1998,183). She notes Lucille Clifton's words:

> I am not done yet. As possible as yeast, as imminent as bread. A collection of safe habits. A collection of cares. Less certain than I seem. More certain than I was. A changed changer. I continue to continue where I have been. Most of my lives is where I'm going. (Tarpley 1998, 1).

Along with the medical components of self-care, African American women also desire to find ways to accept and enhance their physical beauty. Ayana Byrd and Akiba Solomon recognize that in this challenge, African American women have a variety of skin complexions, hair textures, body shapes, career goals, and personal dreams, and are still being challenged in maintaining health care in the following areas: skin, hair, vision and dental (Byrd and Solomon 2005, 10,39).

Skin Care

Susan Taylor teaches that interactive skin care maintenance workshops supply knowledge on skin types, explain the importance of daily cleansing, and reveal the common skin challenges for women of dark complexion (Taylor 2003, 25). Villarosa and Taylor both offer skin care tips as one example of support designed for African American women. Their tips include gentle face cleansing twice a day with oil-free-skin-care products; eating nutritional meals; maintaining stable pigmentation by wearing sunscreen (SPF 15); detecting keloids through knowledge of family history, and scheduling dermatologist appointments to check for dermatosis (dark growth that is visual on the face and neck) and Vitiligo (destruction of melanocytes due to loss of pigment). Villarosa and Taylor concur that by offering African American women insight about the various cleansing techniques and the common skin challenges for women of dark complexion, they were better able to accept skin tones as a blessing from God, overcoming negative messages of inferiority spoken through racism and discrimination (Villarosa1994, 18; Taylor 2003, 25).

As an example, in her skin care lectures, model Beverly Johnson revealed that during her "self-professed junk-food addiction modeling days she looked tired and her complexion tone was poor" (Johnson 1994, 51). Johnson confessed that to maintain good skincare and a high energy level, she had to change her diet from junk food (pastries with white sugar) and diet soda to healthier snacks (fresh fruits, and vegetable trays) and herbal tea. Johnson's example is one in which s prominent woman of color shares her personal experience in an area of self-care, making that information accessible to other women (Johnson 1994, 51).

Hair Care

Taylor explains how the African American women tried to overcome following hair care challenges: styling, growing, and wearing (Taylor 2003, 82). Self-identity that revolved around society's definition of "good hair" has often caused African American women to not respect or appreciate their God-given hair texture, described as kinky, curly, or wavy. Hair care has challenged, frightened, and discouraged African American women from styling, growing, and wearing their own hair. Cosmetic conspiracy through hair straightening tools was adopted for women of African descent. Taylor says that African American women altered hair styles based on the advice of licensed Caucasian cosmetologists who lacked education and knowledge on African hair care (Taylor 2003, 82).

As Pamela Ferrell explains, the rebirth of black pride and the militant black power movement (mid 1960s) promoted a natural hair style called the Afro (Ferrell 1996, 20). The woman of African descent began to embrace self-respect through the acceptance of her natural hair texture. Ferrell comments that pride and self-respect through hair styling was generated through the "I am black and I'm proud" era (Ferrell 1996, 20). This respect for self-began to permeate throughout African American generations, as women began to accept their hair texture and selective style (virgin, relaxed or permed). No longer was their hair defined by the opinion of others. Ferrell, a natural hair care specialist encouraged African American women to stop complying with the "self-defeating cycle of trying to please others" through their hair styles (Ferrell 1996, 51).

Ferrell adds that African American are still dealing with unhealthy hair care, even though professional African American hair stylists have begun to circulate salon and home hair care advice (Ferrell 1996, 60). She makes the following suggestions: First, African American women should make daily affirmation statements. Second, African American women should educate themselves on the various hair conditions for their hair texture. Third, in the evening, she should engage in examination for hair loss or damage. Fourth, the woman of color needs to learn the appropriate care for each hair style in relation to her hair condition. Fifth, education on proper nutrition and nourishment for their hair is of benefit (Ferrell 1996,99).

Ferrell wrote that nutritional food is the key component of healthy hair, as vitamin and minerals (calcium, chlorine, fluorine, sulphur, iodine, iron, magnesium, manganese, phosphorus, potassium, silicon, and sodium) are needed to combat deterioration, disease, and illness. She suggests that the ongoing consumption of fruits and vegetables provides the fuel required to maintain strength in the hair (Ferrell 1996, 101).

Cheryl Talley Moss suggests that African American women must patiently seek guidance on how to self-style without damaging their hair, believing that women should not become co-dependent on a hairdresser (Moss 1999, 38). She teaches how self-confidence can be initiated through learning hair basics such as mirror observation (every angle), shampoo, comb-out, blow-dry, smoothing out hair edges, and controlling frizzles. She believes that African American professional hairstylists can educate African American women that their healthy hair can be attractively styled, can be manageable, and can reveal their self-assurance as African American women, as a woman's physical beauty is transparent through her unique hairstyle, radiant skin and healthy body image (Moss 1999, 38).

To summarize, Mitchem, Hill, and Smith agree that physical health care is important and a necessity for African American women to maintain healthy lifestyles. Taylor, Johnson, and Villarosa understand that women can accept and appreciate their skin tone through the awareness that their complexions are blessing from God. Hair care challenges for African American women can be dealt with as they overcome society's definition and respect their God-given hair texture and style, according to Ferrell. Yet even with these understandings, the African American woman can still struggle with accepting and appreciating her body image.

Body Mass

Millions of Black women of all ages and sizes take advantage of many health benefits of exercise by running, playing tennis, swimming, dancing, taking aerobics classes, walking, and participating in many other sports activities. Nonetheless, many of us don't exercise at all. In fact, Black women are less likely to exercise than white women and Black men. We have a variety of reasons, many of which sound valid, including "I don't know how," "I don't have anyone to watch my children," "I'm too fat," "I'm too old," "I'm tired," or "I don't have access to facilities" (Villarosa 1994, 34).

As will be explored in this section, McCloud, Villarosa and Leonard Jack agree that African American women are often stereotyped as being overweight and living sedentary lifestyles. This stereotype is grounded in reality for many women, causing serious medical problems, especially as long-term obesity leads to chronic diseases (McCloud 2010, 35; Villarosa 1994, 35; Jack 2010, 27). The American Heart Association lists the primary cause of chronic disease (heart, diabetes, high blood pressure, and high cholesterol) as obesity. Richard Cotton and Richard Goldstein adds that obesity increases the risk of type 2 diabetes and cardiovascular diseases (Cotton and Goldstein 1993, 334).

While obesity is a concern, unhealthy weight diagnoses were placed on African American women due to the calculation from Body Mass Index and Waist Circumference used for the Caucasian and European population. According to Lear Scott, Karen Humphries, Simi Kohl, and Laird Birmingham, these calculations do not give an accurate measurement for multicultural populations (Scott, Humphries, Kohl, and Birmingham 2007). A Body Mass Index of 30 and Waist Circumference of 36 are normal for African American women. Carolyn Richardson, Mary Hartley, and Amy Norton note that while African American women are medical healthy at that BMI and waist circumference, Caucasian women with the same measurement are at a greater health risk for diabetes, high blood pressure, and high cholesterol (Richardson and Hartley 2011, 2; Norton 2011, 1).

African American women tend to have more muscle mass and less "visceral fat" (fat around their organs) says Felicia Wade, who recognizes that four aspects should be considered when determining body mass index for African American women (Wade 2014). First, the Body Mass Index's discrepancies may occur due to the dissimilarities in bone mineral content, the density of lean mass, and one's hydration state. Second, an African American woman's body fat may not indicate being overweight or obese if calculations are based on the Body Mass Index of Caucasian women. Finally, the Body Mass Index's overweight threshold for African American women is estimated at 35 which exceed the "medical definition" of less than 25 (Wade 2014).

With a body shape often labeled as curvy with a wide frame, the body type of African American women (the norm) does not always conform to the "white society's ideal body weight" and dress sizes (Cash and Pruzinsky 2002, 234). Understanding the Body Mass Index in relation to the body type of African American women can help them accept themselves. This knowledge can equip them to select dress attire that is appropriate for their shape. Naomi Sims is an advocate of the position that the African American woman's style of dress (personal or professional) should symbolize her femininity and womanhood (Sims 1982, 237). Both Annette Lynch and Kate Betts express how clothing reveals one's self-identity and self-respect (Lynch 1999,116; Betts 2011,10).

As a contemporary example, when Michelle Obama (the first African American first lady of the United States from 2008-2016) chose a fashion statement to compliment her body shape, she motivated African American women to be proud of their curves, Crystal McCrary and Nathan Williams explain (McCrary and Williams 2012, 240). Obama's wardrobe represented her beliefs, family values, and lifestyle choices. McCray and William provide other examples, such as scholars and activists Angela Y. Davis, Essence magazine editor Susan L. Taylor, poet Maya Angelou, and model Naomi Sims, who have also expressed that dignity, pride, and strength are revealed through the clothing selection of African American women (McCrary and Williams 2012, 240).

Andrew Weil believes that even though their fashion may accent the African American women's curves, their physical bodies were often deteriorating from lack of exercise, nutrition, rest, and personal time (Weil 2012, 40). Even though making time for personal fitness routines has been an ongoing challenge for African American women who daily balance their schedules between family responsibilities, career commitments, and communities-care services, physical fitness helps them maintain sharpness of mind, healthy bones, and strong lean muscles (Weil 2012, 40).

Richard Swenson's suggestion on how to restore margin within one's physical activity provides guidance to incorporate fitness work-outs into weekly schedules. When a woman's daily activities lacked physical movements due to desk jobs, health issues, or laziness, this exercise prescription provided a counter attack to a sedentary lifestyle, as developing a loving relationship with her body enhances a person's self-esteem, self-respect, and self-appreciation (Swenson 2004, 108). Natalie Tobert states that sufficient exercise integrates an African American woman's physical abilities with her mental well-being while minimizing the following health risks: inherited chronic diseases, negative society images, and suppressing self-images (Tobert 2017, 86).

Writing of the health benefits of exercise, Dean Ornish and Caldwell Esselstyn explain that moderate to vigorous exercise can lower the risk of developing diabetes, strokes, heart failures, and attacks of exhaustion (Ornish 2008, 42; Esselstyn 2008, 126). Mladen Golubic, a physician from the Disease Reversal Department within the Cleveland Clinic Foundation, indicates that throughout the country, there are free fitness educational courses, lectures, books, and workshops that offer health education tools to African American women. Some of the ways to retrieve the free health resources are through public libraries, free clinics, the internet, community outreach programs, religious institutes, medical plans, and employment offices (McCloud and Ebron 2003, 404). The wellness information explains body composition, offers exercise plans, and gives ideas on how to include fitness fees into an African American woman's family budget. It reminds them that the African American woman's body is energized from exercise.

Taylor notes that nutrition also plays a role in body image and fitness. "Vitamin D, crucial for human health, is found within various foods as well as sunshine. Yet, this and other nutrients are often missing from our diets" (Taylor 2003, 126), and the daily food intake of African American women often lacks sufficient water consumption and a balance of nutrients such as carbohydrates, proteins, and fats (Taylor 2003, 126). Some of the nutritional challenges come through the food choices made. Tracey McQuirter and George Smith recognize the role of Soul Food, the African American cultural meal, as a standard family traditional dinner that raises nutritional concerns. Originating during slavery (in 1800s), it was known as the African American's survival food (unhealthy leftovers) (Smith 2001, 12; McQuirter 2010, 2).

This traditional way of eating, the influence of food advertisements, fast pace lifestyles, and limited income often dictated diet style, as African American women tend to cling to their traditional high-salt, high-fat, and high-cholesterol diet (soothing comfort food), resulting in eating disorders, health issues, and personal insecurities (Smith 2001, 12). Robyn McGee and U-Shaka Craig concur that African American women can reclaim their self-identity, can eliminate unhealthy generational food choices, and can maintain healthier lifestyles by incorporating the educational goals from advocates such as Elijah Muhammad the leader of the Nation of Islam, Malcolm X, a human rights activist, and Dick Gregory a comedian and civil rights activist, who spoke against soul food diets (McGee 2005, 20; Craig 2013, 53).

These traditional food ritual (soul food), women's personal dynamics, institutional practices, physical environment, and family history have led to health problems such as diabetes, cancer, obeslty, and cardiovascular disease (Villarosa 1994, 56). She indicates how alternatives recipes to soul food began to become more popular, as in the mid-1960s, African American restaurant owners began to serve traditional foods that were low in calories, replacing such things as salt pork with chicken stock and using cholesterol-free margarine instead of butter (Villarosa 1994,56). As another health initiative, in 2013 the Library of Congress provided information on how nutritious alternatives for unhealthy recipes have been developed through cookbooks for African Americans, and grant funded health and wellness educational courses, free community culinary classes, and interaction cooking classes have been created (Library of Congress 2013, African History and Cultural; Committee on Diet and Health 1989, 564). While overcoming the traditional food habits is an ongoing process within the African American society, there are many resources available to assist in this process.

To summarize this section, generationally, African American women still are struggling with healthy body image, engaged in an ongoing battle with being stereotyped as overweight since the Body Mass Index caters to Caucasian women. Sims, McCray and Williams indicate that clothing fashion and styles do not enhance the shapes and curves of an African American woman's body. Finally, Lynch and Betts add that African American women's bodies are deteriorating from lack of physical exercise, nutrition, rest and personal time.

Summary

For an African American woman to maintain an energetic lifestyle while engaging in her daily activities, she must be literate in terms of her health. African American women can be guided to healing, health, and wholeness by relying upon their acceptance, understanding and integration of these healthier choices into their everyday lifestyle choices. Her spirit, soul, and body can represent the Messiah when she selectively chooses to maintain a holistic lifestyle balance within these three wellness components: using her faith and dedication to Christ to pursue her ongoing personal relationship with Jesus Christ, utilizing God's word to monitor her emotions, and avoiding physical health problems by maintaining a healthy body composition.

Chapter Four will describe the design, procedure, grant funding, marketing and advertisement, and assessment used for this impact workshop as the Diva's Lifestyle Identity Journey that was created and implemented by the author.

CHAPTER FOUR

DESIGN, PROCEDURE, AND ASSESSMENT

The purpose for this project was to impact the healthcare of women within the Union-Miles community in Cleveland, Ohio by providing six weeks of holistic workshops that help participants integrate God's Divine Wellness plan into their daily lives. This project was designed to promote total wellness and to inspire women of all ages to maintain healthy lifestyles. This was accomplished through their participation within fashion, through modeling, through the daily assigned Scripture readings, and through practicing skills that fostered self-identity awareness. I designed this six week small group experience to illustrate how a Bible-based wellness plan helps to strengthen, motivate, and educate the healthcare choices of African American women in the following holistic areas: spiritual, physical, emotional, mental, vocational, intellectual, and social. Quantitative pre-test and post-test assessment tools including a Likert scale were used to measure the program's effectiveness.

The project consisted of weekly sessions that were held for three hours each day over the course of six weeks, with topical workshops that focused on holistic lifestyle development. Topics such as true self-identity, stress management, relaxation meditations, and fitness tips (cardiovascular exercises and nutrition) were addressed. The workshops offered spiritual growth studies through soul searching. These interactive classes helped the participants to recognize their vocational purpose in relation to their dream careers, and aided them in developing their social skills through communication. The anger management sessions helped them to overcome and control their temper.

The workshops, entitled Diva's Lifestyle Identity Journey and developed by myself, incorporated the following goals:

1. To impact the participants' personal lifestyle through obedience to God's word.

2. To impact the participants' personal lifestyle through exercise.

3. To impact the participants' personal lifestyle through food nourishment.

4. To impact the participants' personal lifestyle through stress management.

5. To impact the participants' holistic lifestyle through their relationships.

6. To impact the participants' personal lifestyle through soul-searching.

After the six sessions, a free community fashion show for the graduates of the project was given in recognition of each participants' inward and outward declaration of knowing who they are in Christ. Finally, there was on-line follow-up which evaluated the outcomes of the workshops within the daily activities of the participants.

Context

Over thirty years, the Lord has led me to women that I could help on their earthly journey while they were seeking God's wellness plan for their lives. Working in the healthcare industry, I have noticed how African American women suffered from the reoccurrence of unhealthy living practices. This appeared to be due to an imbalance of choices that included spiritual, physical, intellectual, emotional, mental, financial, and vocational behaviors. Through building trust in conversation, surveys, and workshops, I learned that the health choices made by African American women were either voluntarily or due to disempowerment.

The ongoing cycle of doctor visits, emotional upheaval, depression, low self-esteem, malnutrition, eating disorders, and revisiting the unemployment office characterized the lifestyle of many of the African American women I met. The African American women who confessed Christianity were wavering in their faith as they endured their daily trials and tribulation. It was not that they did not believe in God's resurrection power; it was that they did not know how to stay rooted in biblical doctrine regardless of their life's daily forecast.

Participants

Ten African American women participated in the Diva's Lifestyle Identity Journey interactive workshop. The participants ranged from eighteen to eighty years of age. They were all beautiful and uniquely made within God's image. Each woman of color had her own dress style, marital status, social skills, skin tone, hair texture, medical issues, family values, church membership, and vocational choice. Their educational level varied from high school graduates to certified trade persons and university graduates. Of the ten participants, two were retired. One participant was a volunteer youth teacher, one a pastor, two financial accountants, one professional hair stylist, an artist, a community leader, and a civil rights activist. Their church ministries varied from pastoral care staff members, worship leaders, elders, trustees, lay persons, to Sunday school teachers.

The African American women testified to being believers in God's Word from five to more than twenty years. They all stated that they were practicing some of what they understood to be God's wellness plan; yet they were challenged in balancing principles of healthy living from Scripture into their daily lifestyles. The African American women stated that when they were faced with difficult circumstances their faith wavered.

The participants were selected through on-line and phone-in registration. The first ten who met the enrollment qualifications were registered. They collectively committed to promptly attend all six sessions. The participants brought their expectations for wellness to the classes, indicating that they were willing to follow the rules and guidelines for the classes.

Procedures

The Diva's Lifestyle Identity Journey small group interactive workshops were designed based on the Bible-based principle that God's wellness plan motivates, encourages, and permits His people to worship and serve Him through their holistic lifestyle. The scriptural foundation was rooted in the following passages: Proverbs 31: 10-31 and Colossians 3: 1-17. A sample of the material utilized is included in the Appendix.

The weekly sessions were held in a private room within the Union Miles Community Center public library. The Diva's Lifestyle Identity Journey workshop was designed for African American women within the community who self-identified as Christian. The enrollment policy was not based on denominations, religious traditions or human religious practice. This openness provided the women with an atmosphere of comfort, security, and peace versus entering an environment of fear, turmoil, and judgment.

Participants were found through a strategic method of marketing and advertisement. Funding was secured, and brochures and flyers were circulated throughout Cleveland's Ward 2 to find participants. Before circulating information on the free community workshop, I had to contact the appropriate parties and organization. I developed rapport with the following non-profit organizations and leadership within Ward 2: community centers, public libraries, recreational locations, inner city women's church's ministries, the Ward 2 councilman, the Salvation Army, and women's shelter home. My family business, Wonderfully Made Inc. (business for profit) and Sassy Ladies Boutique (business for profit) formed a non-profit organization called Esther International. The project was granted funding through Neighborhood Connection, Cleveland Ohio. With the funding, Diva's Lifestyle Identity Journey, a free community outreach program for African American women, was developed.

Before classes began, Esther International's committee met weekly on Thursday for two hours. The focus of the meetings was on preparations for the upcoming interactive workshops. The meeting opened with prayer for personal goals, family members and the success of the project. We discussed marketing and advertising strategies, and I gave weekly updates on our contact list, distributions of our brochures and flyers, advertising our upcoming free community outreach class sessions. I also discussed the progress on the facilitator's manual and participants' handout.

The facilitator's manual was designed to simplify class format and to train future instructors. This instructor's manual provided the following class information: registration package, brochure sample, attendance sheets, class sessions, detailed notes on various subjects discussed, and samples of pre-test and post-test surveys.

Handout packages offered participants the necessary information, a journal, pencil, weekly discussion information, weekly homework assignments, Diva's proclamation, *Our Daily Bread 90-day* edition, congratulation certificate, and a six-week agenda. Weekly words of encouragement were offered through group emails and posted on our Facebook account.

The ten women participated in six sessions that instructed them how to implement God's holistic living skills into their daily activities according to the prepared curriculum outline. The wellness program challenged and encouraged them to discover, accept, and appreciate their most important asset, themselves in Christ. The interactive workshops helped the women to remain rooted in Christ by applying the Scriptures during economic challenges. To help improve their overall health and wellbeing, the classes taught them how to unify their spirit with their soul and bodies.

Each workshop began with prayer, relaxation meditation, and the following Diva's proclamation:

I am strong! I have been and will continue to be. I am happy! I do not depend on others to make me happy. I am in a daily pursuit of fulfilling my purpose and that makes me happy. I am successful! I have achieved by leaps and bounds in my life and there are many more to come in the future! I am amazing! I am good enough, beautiful and a wonderful person. Most of all, I LOVE ME (Esther International, In and Out).

This declaration was spoken out loud as they looked at themselves in a mirror. The purpose was to remind them that their spoken words have power. The statement was a declaration in faith about their identity in Christ.

The Diva's decorum (proclamation) was given during each group session. It was important for each woman to develop trust as they shared their private and personal concerns with each other. Every session, the participants made their commitment to respect shared information, to watch voice tone, and to practice active listening skills.

Every interactive meeting offered a stress release exercise. Soft inspirational music was played. Tai Chi, 3 R's, chair yoga, or devotional readings were implemented to initiate a peaceful atmosphere. Before each relaxation session, participants were reminded to listen to their body and to prayerfully seek to be led by the Holy Spirit. During this time, the women were encouraged to let go of their concerns, hectic schedules, to do lists, or missed opportunities. This was their time to rejuvenate and prepare for their wellness journey, individually and collectively.

In each session, I read one of the assigned devotions from the *Our Daily Bread 90-Day sample edition*, which was handed out in the first session. I prayerfully selected a day that coincided with the weekly topics. The homework assignments helped them to incorporate consistent Bible reading for their spiritual self-development and interaction time with God.

Nutrition information for their soul and body was offered throughout the sessions. Traditional family meals were reviewed and altered for healthier choices. Educational sections on vitamins and supplements consistent with their individual physician's recommendations were discussed. A suggested nutrition fact sheet was handed out. This fact sheet listed the various vitamins and food choices that may prevent or treat chronic diseases. They were encouraged to check with their physician before taking any supplements or vitamins.

Healthy snacks were distributed during each session. The participants were required to journal when they used the healthy eating tips which were presented throughout the workshops. Re-evaluation of their food selections were recorded weekly. Food choices were examined through family tradition, cravings, and healthy and unhealthy choices.

Every class had homework assignments and journaling exercises. Journal entries were designed to help them to understand what was going on internally in relation to their spirit, soul and body. Writing was intended to help them to experience their unique emotional journey. It assisted them in their reflection upon the following recording progress: brain-storming, making decisions, and noting successes. As the facilitator, I reviewed their journals weekly and offered prayer suggestions based on scriptures, which assisted them on their Diva's Lifestyle Identity Journey.

Each session ended with a question and answer period. I encouraged each woman to take advantage of our intimate times together. They were given the opportunity to offer personal reflections and ask questions. I reminded them that their sharing blessed the other women in the class who may be struggling or were afraid to ask a question. Strict confidentiality was enforced.

I Know Who I Am (Sinach, 2012) was the dismissal song. Its lyrics and creative physical movements energized the women's spirits and reminded them of who they were in Christ and in relation to self, family, and community. This Bible-based song brought God's words to life within their souls, allowing them to declare and decree their identity in Christ regardless of their circumstances.

The first week's class was the orientation. It started with a stress release meditation. The women were greeted and welcomed. This friendly invitation permitted them to experience peace in Christ as they shared their fitness concerns, health fears, personal goals, emotional hurts, and disappointments. On this day, I discussed the compassion and desires of my wellness ministry. I discussed my ministry and the potential impact to their healthcare through my God-given creative, educational, motivational, and fashion styles.

The remaining time in that first session was spent on stress awareness. A stress evaluation clarified areas of anxiety and offered several tension relief remedies. The breathing breaks were to be implemented at work when they felt overwhelmed. The 3 R's stress release exercise brought inner calmness.

Week two focused on identity crisis. Each woman wore her favorite jewelry or outfit that reflected her personality for that day. This was designed to help illustrate how important it is to understand one's current emotional state. The women reflected on the reason for the attachment to the item or clothing. This was planned to help them redefine their lifestyle by evaluating their self-perception and the perception of others, and to evaluate their self-confidence throughout their seasons of life (menopause, health issues, financial difficulties, relationship drama, self-worth). This time of sharing provided some insight on their self-worth, self-acceptance, and self-observation.

A self-identity check list was distributed to encourage each African American woman to see herself through the eyes of Christ. The workshop suggested tips on accepting constructive criticism versus accepting people's negative opinions about them. The journal exercise on viewpoints of self-image was implemented. A period of twenty minutes was given to all of them to express, through writing, their responses towards the compliments and criticism they received in the past week, allowing them to weigh remarks given and received against God's thoughts of themselves (the foundation for self-esteem and identity).

Week three addressed the topic of healthy heart and soul. The soul-searching exercise was designed to reveal to each woman her life purpose, self-accomplishments, and affirmation for her lifestyle changes. The mind check list helped the women to identify their thought patterns, to develop mind strengthening exercises, and to assist them to include nutritional snacks (mind food). Soul voice identification led to soul toning through spiritual prayers.

Lament Prayer formation and journaling exercises were used in this session to soul search and authentically express their true feelings and to release them to God. This session demonstrated that they do have control over what thoughts they pondered on. The class reminded the women that removing negative thoughts is an ongoing process. This session reminded and encouraged them to renew their minds daily in Gods' word.

Week four educated the women in the areas of body image and fitness. This interactive session exposed the negative self-body image they may have formed from the distorted view society placed on them as African American women. The scriptural teaching on being fearfully and wonderfully made was used to diminish their images of low self-esteem and a lack of sexual attractiveness, and to acknowledge and seek help with their eating disorders. The explanations of the African woman's curvy shape helped them understand why certain styles were fashionable on them. The chronic disease session explained warning signs, effects, risk factors and prevention tools. An acceptance of their blessed bodies was encouraged to enhance their self-esteem, self-value and self-worth.

The components of fitness were discussed and illustrated during an interactive work-out session, using Zumba movements for cardiovascular exercise, with a strength training focus on abdominals and legs. Fredifit Pilate was also used to illustrate core flexibility. Exercise prescriptions were given to assure that they maintained their physical fitness. Scriptures related to fitness were incorporated into their daily confessions.

Week five focused on maintaining control of spoken words, by affirming the importance of words, providing conversation tips, and exploring the concept of using a Christ-like speaking principle. A speaking checklist was also used that asked: Is it necessary? Is it true? Is it loving? Is It Scriptural?

Journaling of their word choices was recommended to reveal habitual word choices, and a seven-day mouth fast was encouraged to aid them with the elimination process of a negative word choices. In this mouth fast, for seven days the participants would not speak words or phrases that caused negative outcomes within their daily activities, and they were to record the outcome of the words spoken within their journals.

Week six addressed dress attire, considering how dressing for success in every area of their lives can motivate the African American women to take pride in their fashion statements. The slogan used was "whatever you wear should reflect the real you." This section emphasized that dress style has power, just like the spoken word, and represents a powerful image of self-identity. Dress attire games were played which expressed the importance of colors in relation to mood swings.

The sixth session concluded with the Diva's Lifestyle Fashion Show Graduation. The women illustrated who they were through the three fashion styles:

creative, career, and classic. Each woman selected the styles that expressed her self-identity at home, work, school, and displayed them in a ballroom social event. The audience was astounded and expressed admiration as they watched each woman walk the runway with boldness, style, and in radiance. Each time they elegantly walked, they proclaimed "I Know Who I Am."

Because motivation can be a struggle for any self-improvement type of activity, these interactive workshops gave the African American women various incentives to be used as ongoing health and wellness motivators. Healthy snacks were served weekly. Esther International In/Out's Facebook site posted the following: weekly words of encouragement, holistic blogs, class reminders, prayer request, and uplifting and inspiration success stories. Upon completion of the impact workshop each woman was given a piece of jewelry of her choice and a congratulatory card.

Assessment

Two questionnaires were distributed for the project assessment. The first questionnaire was given at the beginning of the orientation session. It had eighteen quantitative questions designed to measure the project goals. The participants evaluated each question using a scale from one to seven; (1), strongly disagree, (2), moderately disagree (3), slightly disagree (4), neither agree nor disagree (5), slightly agree (6), moderately agree and (7), strongly agree. At the end of six weeks, the second questionnaire was given. It had the same eighteen statements given at the beginning with the addition of three qualitative questions regarding overall experience. This assessment is included in Appendix II, and the results of this project and assessment tool are discussed in Chapter Five.

CHAPTER FIVE

REPORTING THE RESULTS

The design and procedure of the project were described in Chapter Four. The purpose for this project was to impact the healthcare of women within the Union-Miles community in Cleveland, Ohio by providing six weeks of holistic workshops that helped the participants integrate God's Divine Wellness Plan into their daily lives. The research question is: what impact will this six weeks of holistic workshops have on the healthcare of the women within the Union-Miles community in Cleveland, Ohio?

This chapter reports the results of the assessment statements and discusses the qualitative responses to the open-ended questions which gave further details on how the Diva's Lifestyle Identity Journey project impacted the participants' lifestyle choices. The composite score for each goal and the average result for each pre-and post-assessment statement will be reviewed.

The responses of the ten participants (n=10) who completed the six weeks of wellness sessions were the ratings indicators. The statements were based on a Likert agreement scale as follows: 1 = strongly disagree, 2= moderately disagree, 3 = slightly disagree, 4 = neither agree nor disagree, 5 = slightly agree, 6 = moderately agree, 7 = strongly agree.

The arranged order of the goals in this chapter are from the results of the quantitative answers, with the goals with the highest impact presented first. The subsequent goals will be discussed in the order of their degree of impact. Table 1 lists the average change between the pre-and post-assessment for each goal. This will be the order in which all goals are explained.

This project was effective in measuring the extent to which holistic lifestyle workshops impacted the African American women participants' health and wellness choices. Each goal showed a degree of positive impact. Goal 1 portrayed the highest level of impact, followed by Goal 2.

Table 1: Average Statistical Change by Goals (Greatest to Least)

Goals		Average Change
Health through obedience to God's Word........	Goal 1	1.70
Health through intentional physical activities....	Goal 2	1.10
Health through soul-searching......................	Goal 6	.80
Health through stress management...............	Goal 4	.63
Health through food nourishment..................	Goal 3	.33
Health through self-identity........................	Goal 5	.30

Note: Ten participants provided data for the statements; n=10

Goal 1: Health Through Obedience to God's Word

In this workshop, Goal 1 scored the highest. As stated, the goal was to impact the participants' personal lifestyle through obedience to God's Word. The questions measuring the goal were: (1) I try to live a healthy lifestyle in obedience to God's word (#15); (2) There are specific Scriptures that help me to be obedient to God (#8); (3) Obedience to God's word affects my personal lifestyle (#1).

Table 2: Goal 1: Health Through Obedience to God's Word

Statement	Average			
	Pre-Test	Post-Test	Change	Respondent
(15) Obedience to God's Word affects my personal lifestyle	2.6	6.7	+4.1	10
(8) There are specific Scriptures that help me to be obedient to God	5.5	6.4	+ .9	10
(1) I try to live a healthy lifestyle in obedience to God's Word	6.0	6.1	+ .1	10
Composite	4.7	6.4	+1.7	n=10

Note: Likert Scale: (7), strongly agree, (6), moderately agree, (5), slightly agree, (4), neither agree nor disagree (3), slightly disagree (2), moderately disagree (1), strongly disagree; There were ten participants who provided information for the pre-test and post-test; n=10.

Table two reflects that the wellness workshops were effective in helping the African American women to comprehend the importance of God's word within their faith walk in relation to their healthy lifestyles choices. The change in statement fifteen was +4.1, which showed the African American women's obedience to God's word moved closer to "strongly agree" than to "moderately disagree." During the qualitative questions, the participants concurred that by abiding by God's word, their lifestyle choices were simplified, fulfilling, and stress free.

The change in statement eight was +.9. The impact change moved from "moderately agree" to the "strongly agree range," since the before and after quantitative survey portrayed that specific scriptures helped them to remain within their faith.

The change in statement one remained within the "strongly agree range" with little change. The participants stated that they try to live a lifestyle in accordance with God's Word.

Goal 2: Health Through Intentional Physical Activities

The next goal with the highest prominence had a composite score of 1.16. The participants responded to the following three questions that fundamentally provided the measurement for this goal: (1) I am aware of practical ways that I can increase my daily physical activities (#2); (2) There are certain physical activities that I do because I know they are a part of a healthy lifestyle (#7); (3) I must set aside specific time for exercise in order to be healthy (#14). Table 3 gives the results.

Table 3: Goal 2. Health: Intentional Physical Activities

Statement	Average Pre-Test	Post-Test	Change	Respondents
(2) Practical ways to increase my physical activities	4.2	6.5	+2.3	10
(7) Certain physical movements that I do are a part of a healthy lifestyle	5. 5	6.3	+ .8	10
(14) I must set aside specific time for exercise in order to be healthy	6.1	6.5	+ .4	10
Composite	5.3	6.4	+1.1	n=10

Note: Likert Scale: (7), strongly agree, (6), moderately agree, (5), slightly agree, (4), neither agree nor disagree (3), slightly disagree (2), moderately disagree (1), strongly disagree; There were ten participants who provided information for the pre-test and post-test; n=10

Table 3 illustrates how the African American women in the group received fitness benefits through the physical activity group experience. The change in the score for question two was +2.3, which increased from 4.2 in pre-assessment to 6.5 in the post-assessment. The increase in the score range demonstrated that the African American women collectively increased in knowledge as to possible physical activities they could use within their daily schedule.

In statement seven, the change was +.8. This score represented the participants' realization of the importance to incorporate physical activities within their daily movements. African American women moved from pre-test score of 5.5 to post-test score of 6.3. The score demonstrates a slight change within participants' active lifestyles.

The average participants' score of +.4, was reflected in question fourteen. The pre-test score of 6.1 revealed the participants' acknowledgement of the need to schedule fitness time to live a healthy lifestyle. The post-test average score was 6.5. In the qualitative responses, the participants agreed that the educational component on fitness helped them to understand the health benefits for setting a side time for personal work-out sessions. Several of the participants explained how they now see the connection between sedentary lifestyle and chronic disease.

Goal 6: Health Through Soul Searching

The next goal of prominence was goal 6 which addressed health awareness in the area of personal soul searching. The participants became conscious of their lifestyles responses in relation to their personal feelings and emotional responses to others. The assessment of this goal was carried out using the following statements: (1) I am in touch with my feelings (#12); (2) I understand the feelings behind my actions (#18); (3) My life is well balanced (#6). The purpose for these questions was to impact the participants' awareness to their responses to life situation. The participants stated this session on soul-searching helped them to be more conscious of their feelings and alertness of their emotional response and Bible-based replies. The assessment of the participants' responses follows in table 4.

Table 4: Goal 6. Health: Through Soul Searching

Statement	Average Score			
	Pre-Test	Post-Test	Change	Respondents
(12) I understand the feelings behind my actions	4.9	6.2	1.3	10
(18) my life is well balanced	4.8	5.7	+ .9	10
(6) I am in touch with my feelings	6.0	6.2	+ .2	10
Composite	5.23	6.03	+.8	n=10

Note: Likert Scale: (7), strongly agree, (6), moderately agree, (5), slightly agree, (4), neither agree nor disagree (3), slightly disagree (2), moderately disagree (1), strongly disagree; There were ten participants who provided information for the pre-test and post-test; n=10.

In statement twelve, the change was +1.3. This revealed a movement from "slightly agree" (+4.9) to "strongly agree" (+6.2). The participants expressed through their qualitative comments that their family's religious upbringing aided them in their response of not permitting their feelings to control their lifestyles choices. However, through this impact workshop, the participants stated how the lament prayers and soul-searching homework assignment helped them to develop their personal faith. This assisted them with trusting God in their personal emotional development instead of relying on their families' faith in God.

In statement eighteen, the change was +.9. In their qualitative responses, the participants explained how their awareness increased in the area of the necessity of incorporating me-time. They explained how they were viewing a balance lifestyle from the perspective of taking care of family while working.

The average group score of +.2 was the participants' response to question six. The slight movement from pre-test score of +6.0 to post-test score of +6.2 reflected a slight change in being in touch with their own feelings. The group participants agreed that the soul-searching exercises permitted them to become more in touch with their emotion as they dealt with grief, anxiety, and health challenges.

Goal 4: Health Stress Management

The next goal in prominence was stress management with an average increase of +.63. The participants responded to the following three statements: (1) When life is difficult there are healthy things I do to reduce my stress (#10); (2) When life is stressful, I am able to quiet my mind (#16); (3) During difficult times, I know how to reduce my stress (#4). In the following table 5, the results are posted.

Table 5: Goal 4: Health: Through Stress Management

Statement	Average Score			
	Pre-Test	Post-Test	Change	Respondents
(10) when life is stressful I am able to quiet my mind	5.2	6.2	+ 1.0	10
(16) During difficult times, I know how to reduce my stress	5.3	6.2	+ .9	10
(4) when life is difficult there are healthy things I do to reduce my stress	6.3	6.3	+0.0	10
Composite	5.6	6.23	+ .63	n=10

Note: Likert Scale: (7), strongly agree, (6), moderately agree, (5), slightly agree, (4), neither agree nor disagree (3), slightly disagree (2), moderately disagree (1), strongly disagree; There were ten participants who provided information for the pre-test and post-test; n=10.

In statement ten the change was +1.0. This change indicated a movement from "slightly agree" to "moderately agree". The group's participants reported their awareness of being able to remain calm during stressful times.

In statement sixteen the change was +.9. This change indicated that the pre-test score moved from +5.3 "moderately agree" to +6.2 "strongly agree". The group's participants reported their awareness of the connection between life challenges and the health effects from anxiety attacks. They were affectively educated on the necessity for stress management during difficult times.

There was no change for question four from pre-test to post-test assessment. The group participants' answers to the qualitative question about their stress management group experience revealed the benefits received through their faith declarations. They stated their pre-test score was based on physical relaxation techniques versus spiritual. This revealed wellness through spiritual growth.

Goal 3: Health Through Food Nourishment

The next goal in prominence was nutrition. The participants were asked to give feedback on the following three statements: (1) I understand what makes food healthy (#9); (2) I am aware of how I eat affects my health (#13); and (3) When faced with the choice of healthy and unhealthy food options, I usually choose the healthy option (#3). The results follow in Table 6.

Table 6: Goal 3. Health: Through Food Nourishment

Statement	Average Pre-Test	Post-Test	Change	Respondents
(9) I understand what makes food healthy	5.9	6.4	+ .5	10
(13) I am aware of how I eat affects my health	6.2	6.6	+ .4	10
(3) when faced with the choice of healthy and unhealthy food options, I usually choose the healthy option	5.6	5.7	+ .1	10
Composite	5.9	6.23	+ .33	n=10

Note: Likert Scale: (7), strongly agree, (6), moderately agree, (5), slightly agree, (4), neither agree nor disagree (3), slightly disagree (2), moderately disagree (1), strongly disagree; There were ten participants who provided information for the pre-test and post-test; n=10.

In statement nine, the average score rate of +.5 represented the pre-test score of +5.9 which changed to post-test of +6.4. In the qualitative responses, the participants agreed that the discussions and handouts on vitamins and supplements provided information on nourishment for chronic disease. The participants stated that the nutrition section helped them understand how to prevent obesity and chronic diseases.

Statement thirteen, with an average score increase of +.4, indicated a slight movement from +6.2 to +6.6, and remained within "strongly agree." The group participants stated they had interpreted the question based on their intellectual understanding of the effects of food. However, all ten participants within the qualitative question wrote how the holistic discussion enlightened their understanding on how their nutrition choices affected their total wellbeing (spirit, soul, and body). In statement three, the pre-test score of +5.6 movement to +5.7 was minimal, with the average increase of +.1.

Goal 5: Health Through Self-Identity

The next goal in prominence was self-identity. The assessment for this goal was implemented through the following statements: (1) my relationship with God helps me to feel good about myself #11); (2) when I think about myself, I like what I see (#5); (3) my relationship with those closest to me helps me to feel good (#17). The participants' responses follow, in Table 7.

Table 7: Goal 5. Health Through Self-Identity

Statement	Average Pre-Test	Post-Test	Change	Respondents
(11) when I think about myself I like what I see	5.6	6.2	+ .6	10
(5) My relationship with God helps me feel good about myself	6.5	6.1	+ .4	10
(17) my relationship with those closest to me helps me to feel good	6.6	6.5	- .1	10
Composite	6.23	6.26	.30	n=10

Note: Likert Scale: (7), strongly agree, (6), moderately agree, (5), slightly agree, (4), neither agree nor disagree (3), slightly disagree (2), moderately disagree (1), strongly disagree; There were ten participants who provided information for the pre-test and post-test; n=10.

In statement five, the average group score of +.4 remained within the "strongly agree" category. The participants' score in question eleven was +.6. The movement from pre-test +5.6 to + 6.2, moving from "slightly agree" to "moderately agree." In the qualitative response, the group participants revealed their awareness of negative thoughts about their self-value when their focus is not Christ-centered. Question seventeen's average score rate of -.1 was minimal.

Response to Open Ended Questions

As has already been noted in the specific goals, at the end of the post-test, the participants were given the following three open ended questions to evaluate their overall experience within the Diva's Lifestyle Identity Journey interactive workshops: "List two or three ways that your experience in this group was helpful in making changes in your lifestyles. "List one or two biblical principles you learned during the six weeks' workshop that will or have helped you to develop or maintain a Christ-like character. "List one or two inheritances you recognized have had a strong or weak influence on your lifestyle choices. Each question also asked the participants to explain their answers.

The participants gave a 100% response rate to all the qualitative questions. The participants' answers are tabulated by "key words." The table below is arranged in order of prominence of the three most frequent keywords. The following is a summary of their responses:

Table 8. Helpful Lifestyle Experiences
Question #1 List two or three ways that your experiences in this group were helpful in making changes in your lifestyle. Please explain.

Most commonly used words	Number of Responses N=10
1. Self-acceptance	10
2. Self-appreciation	8
3. Confrontation	7

All ten women stated that they learned self-acceptance of their uniqueness as created in God's image. Eight of the women wrote that they can now appreciate their personalities and body shapes without being intimidated by other women's gifts, talents, and physical appearances. Seven women said that they learned how to confront their fears of vulnerability with women. They stated that some of their female friends betrayed their trust. Going forward they are confident in their trust in God.

Table 9. Biblical Principles Learned
> Question #2 List two biblical principles you learned during this six-week
> workshop that will or has helped you to maintain a Christ-like character.
> Please explain.

	Most
commonly used words	Number of Responses N=10
1. Word conscious	10
2. Humility	9
3. Scripture Passage Proverbs 31:10-31	7

All ten of the women stated that they are more word conscious in relation to death and life in the power of their words (Prov. 18:21). They stated that they noticed that their positive and negative statements manifested within their daily activities; therefore, they needed to speak life versus death. Nine of the women commented on learning how to live holistically in humility through transparency. Seven of the women replied as to how the Scripture passage found within Proverbs 31:10-31 helped them to develop and maintain the Christ-like characters of a virtuous woman. They stated that as they have applied some of the mouth skills learned in the workshop, they have received positive feedback from family members, co-workers, and friends.

Table 10. Cultural Inheritances
> Question #3 List one or two cultural inheritances you recognized that have
> had a strong or weak influence on your lifestyle choices. Please explain.

Most commonly used words	Number of Responses N=10
1. Interaction with men	8
2. Food choices	7
3. Family values	6

Eight of the women stated that their interactions with men have been less controlling, with some comments in the workshops noting that in their families' cultural upbringing the women dominated men, since there were no male role models within their households. Seven women commented that they had to reevaluate their food choices because of their cultural upbringing. Six of the women stated that their cultural inheritance has influenced their lifestyle around family values.

While not statistically measured in this section, within conversations in the workshops and on-line, the participants concluded that the holistic workshops were uplifting, educational, energizing, and creatively fun. Some commented that even though they were familiar with some of the information, it was refreshing to be reminded of the areas they needed to work on. It reminded them to seek restoration through the Holy Spirit's guidance. For example, four of the women knew that their lifestyles were out of balance in the areas of nutrition, personal time with God, and me-time. They stated that the workshop reminded them and gave them some simple solutions on how to maintain balanced lifestyles (spirit, soul, and body).

This chapter gave the results of the six-week holistic lifestyle interactive workshops. In the next chapter, I will reflect upon the project based upon the goals and how this experience has affected me personally.

CHAPTER SIX

SUMMARY AND REFLECTION

It comes in an array of body sizes with a structure capturing other ethnicity eyes. Although in a negative disguise, a black woman's butt was seen as a disgrace. Now look all over the place. You can't escape the other race emulating black woman's shape. Don't make any mistake my bodacious booty is beautifully great. Even before the media decided to appreciate. It is my heritage trait not surgically or artificially created.

My hair is a lace coming in different grades that I can embrace. Its diverse colors are brown, black, gray and hazelnut. Along with a style that compliment my beauty from braids, afro, straight, wool, locks or a fierce cut.

My image and self-esteem is dynamically supreme my blackness has been influenced by many but defined by none. Yet I will not allow negative words about black beauty to be won. Nor portray or distort with degrading images display. However, I will embrace the diverse positive images defined as uniquely divine.

My black is courage validation, self-belief, independent, deserving, happy, beautiful, vigorous, pure, original, love, uplifting, a pearl of wisdom, intelligent, inspiring, enlightening, a goddess and fine. It exemplifies all of me with a rainbow personality that has its own originality. My Black Is Beautiful and ranks High in Principality (*My Black Is Beautiful 3 (Woman)*, Naomi Johnson).

How does an African American woman see herself? From the days of the slave trade, through the Antebellum period, and now into the twentieth-first century, African American women have spoken and written in many ways, defining and redefining their color diversity, heritage traits, body image, professional status, and expressions of self-worth. One example is Naomi Johnson's poem, *My Black Is Beautiful*, which expresses how an African American woman's self-esteem and body image originates through self-portrait.

Picture her description of hair: "My hair is a lace coming in different grades that I can embrace. Its diverse colors are brown, black, gray and hazelnut. Along with a style that compliment my beauty from braids, afro, straight, wool, locks or a fierce cut" (Johnson 2013). Johnson's images serve as a reminder that while there is much that African American women have in common (heritage, history, skin color, hair), within those categories there is a wide variety of experience and expression. It was my hope through this project to motivate, to educate, and to make a Christ-like impact within the lifestyles of African American women, recognizing the common themes of their experiences, and celebrating the diversity of their lives.

This project created and presented six weeks of holistic workshops which assisted the women with developing and maintaining healthy lifestyles throughout their daily activities with the following research question: What impact will this six week holistic workshop have on the healthcare of the women within the Union-Miles community in Cleveland, Ohio?

The results from the workshops revealed that the sessions successfully reached the goals of the project. The participants' feedback through the assessment, ongoing Facebook posts, thank you notes, and referrals showed their gratitude and excitement, and confirmed the positive impact made on their lifestyle choices. The six weeks of holistic interactive workshops successfully exposed the African American women to the Messiah's rules for good physical, mental, and spiritual well-being. The success of the holistic workshops has made a lasting and ongoing impact upon the African American women participants and upon myself, and I am grateful to God for His provision.

In this chapter, I will share my reflections regarding the goals of the project. Second, I will share how I applied the results from the project to my ministry context, and my hope as to how the project might transition into a community program through grant funding. Third, I will offer a few areas for further study. Finally, I will discuss the results of my personal goals that were listed at the beginning of the project.

Project Goals

The following project list is based from the most prominent goal to the least prominent: 1. To impact the participants' personal lifestyle through obedience to God's Word; 2. To impact the participants' personal lifestyle through intentional physical activities; 3. To impact the participants' personal lifestyle through soul-searching; 4. To impact the participants' personal lifestyle through stress management; 5. To impact the participants' personal lifestyle through food nourishment; 6. To impact the participants' lifestyle through self-identity.

Goal Number One
Personal Lifestyle Through Obedience to God's Word

This goal had the largest change, in what was the underlying purpose for the workshop, which was for the African American women to recognize, accept, and know who they are in Christ. I prayerfully designed the workshop to emphasize that the survival and lifestyle of Christian women were anchored in meditation, acceptance, and application of God's word throughout their daily activities.

In the group discussions and the qualitative comments made in the evaluations, the participants expressed how the workshops helped them to transition the spiritual (God's word) into the natural (physical interaction and healthy life choices). For example, the Mouth Trap/Word Choices workshop offered insight through examination of word choices. Taking inventory of their word choices helped them understand the various positive and negative outcomes from self-talk and the feedback of others. The participants stated that the mouth prescription homework assignment helped them to control their tongues through being silent, fasting, having a partner accountability, and accepting the responsibility of cleaning up their word choices and apologizing when needed.

Reflecting back over the session, the participants and I were grateful for the Old and New Testament passages used within the workshop. Prov.31:26, "She speaks with wisdom, and faithful instruction is on her tongue," and Col. 3:17a, "And whatever you do, whether in word or deed, do it all in the name of the Lord Jesus," encouraged us and helped us to see how our characters and behavior patterns revealed our personal identities in Christ. This was made possible when we chose to live out God's Word within our spirits and bodies.

Goal Number Two

Personal Lifestyle Through Intentional Physical Activities

The next finding in prominence, with a composite increase of 1.6, was in the category of an awareness and recognition of African American women's unique body images and physiques, and their maintenance through intentional physical activities. After the Body Image and Fitness workshop, the participants' receptiveness to the Body Mass Index information was illustrated through the following: their new way of purchasing clothing, their fashion style, and their willingness to share the Body Mass Index information with other African American.

The exercise component of each workshop session catered to the curvy shape body type. The group participants stated that the work-out helped them as curvaceous shape women to tone and sculpt their body images, to maintain energy level, to feel comfortable within their own body, and to feel good about their physical appearances. The homework included the verse from Ps. 139:14a, "I praise you because I am fearfully and wonderfully made," which was incorporated as reassurance to the African American women that their unique and beautiful bodies are used to praise and reverence God.

Looking back over the body image workshop, this new insight about African American women's body composition instilled self-confidence in them about their physical appearance. Also, this session motivated and encouraged me to continue my daily exercise routines and Scripture proclamations. This inspired me to continue to instruct African American women about dress style and fashion for curvy women while also assisting them in soul-searching.

Goal Number Six
Personal Lifestyle Through Soul-Searching

The third prominent finding was in the area of soul-searching. Even though this ranked third, the participants reported how the Healthy Heart/Soul workshop class helped them to be more soul conscious in relation to their feelings and emotions. By basing their lifestyles responses (personal and professional) on God's Word, they did not allow their behaviors to reflect their feelings of jealousy, anger, rage, malice, greed, or evil desires (Col. 3: 7-9).

The participants stated that by applying the soul-searching homework assignment throughout their week, they had new awareness to their decisions made through self-deception. The soul-searching assignment helped them recognize and accept an honest inward examination of their feelings and to identify the various voices within their souls (God, self, or Satan). For example, the participants stated that the journaling homework allowed them opportunities to record their emotional state and situations that led to the various feelings. The lament prayer guided them on how to pray to God about their soul's deep hurts, angers, betrayals and fears.

Reflecting back over the Healthy Heart/Soul session, it was reassuring to be told by the participants that through soul-searching, Scripture references were now a part of their spiritual foundation for healthy living on earth. The African American women were seeking lifestyle wisdom from God's word versus society and family traditions. The women stated that they were not making as many unhealthy choices in spiritual, physical, mental, emotional, financial, vocational, and intellectual areas. The lament prayers helped the group participants and myself to recognize, accept, and acknowledge our feelings throughout our lifestyles and environment. This motivated me to continue to educate women within the Union and Miles area about God's wellness plan for them.

Goal Number Four
Personal Lifestyle Through Stress Management

The next prominent goal was recognizing the role of stress management. Ranking fourth, with a composite score of .68, the women did acknowledge the value of stress management. The group participants informed me that stress release exercises that were used as coping instruments helped them to respond to the following life challenges in a less stressful way: threatening situations, disappointments, grief, promotions, and financial difficulties. They stated that they used the following techniques when they felt stressful, which released some of their anxieties: The Tai Chi and rest relaxation (3 R's) exercise, Scripture references on peace, breathing techniques, and gentle movements. The Scripture reference used was Col.315: "Let the peace of Christ rule in your hearts, since as members of one body you were called to peace. And be thankful." Participants stated how refreshed they felt after engaging in the stress exercises before going to work, attending business meetings, or dealing with conflict at work or home. They stated they used the journal entries to document their progress. Participants stated that throughout the day, the inspirational message placed on Facebook helped them to endure the various circumstances they encountered within their work or home environment.

Reflecting back over the stress release sessions, the participants' acknowledgements on how the stress release exercises, Scripture references journaling assignments, and inspirational messages posted on Facebook inspired them as well as myself to maintain our stress levels. This finding encouraged me to continue educating African American women and myself about the various Bible-based stress management tools that can help us handle stress and to detoxify stressors; yet, more understanding was needed in the area of emotional stress release.

Goal Number Three

Personal Lifestyle Through Food Nourishment

The next prominent goal was a lifestyle improvement through a healthier perspective on food nourishment. The two statements regarding improved understanding of nutritional information showed a .5 and .4 increase, but only a .1 increase was reported in regards to any difference in what food choices the women make. However, the qualitative question as well as verbal comments in the workshops indicated that there was a good understanding that their food intake could cause emotional outburst, health issues, and ongoing chronic diseases through general inheritance. The women also expressed their gratitude in being able to implement the following food nourishment skills into their traditional meals: 1. Learning how to cook foods that prevent obesity and chronic; conditions; 2. Being able to recognize and avoid food intake for emotional comfort; and 3. Being able to use healthier food substitutions for their families' traditional meals which they inherited.

The African American women stated that the healthy snacks served, the instruction provided on what makes food healthy, and an increased awareness of their food intake helped them to make better food choices and prevent chronic diseases. Through online comments, the group participants noted how they are taking their snacks and lunches to work versus grabbing snacks from the vending machine at work or purchasing sandwiches from fast food restaurants.

The participants also reported how evening journaling about their emotional state and food choices revealed a pattern of unhealthy food intake. In order not to be consumed with guilt, they used and found comfort in the following techniques learned: they sought God through lament prayer, they verbally stated that "I have taken off the old self with its practices and have put on the new self, which is renewed in knowledge in the image of its Creator" (Col. 3: 9b-10), and they sang the theme song "I Know Who I Am".

The group participants' feedback from the qualitative question number three indicated that the cooking tips learned helped them to reevaluate food choices made based on their cultural upbringing. They expressed their appreciation on being able to continue to cook and pass on their family's traditional meals in a healthy and more nutritional way. Reflecting back, the food nourishment session educated the group participants and reminded me of the health benefits for eating nutritionist foods.

Goal Number Five

Personal Lifestyle Through Self-Identity

The next prominent goal was through self-identity. The average group score remained within the "strongly agree" category, with the greatest increase, .6, in the statement, "when I think about myself I like what I see." The group participants shared that they were aware of their self-acceptance of negative thoughts about their self-worth at various times in their lives, and that negative view of themselves had resulted in low self-esteem and a defeating self-image. The women also stated that the Identity session helped them to develop and maintain their self-worth and self-esteem in Christ, affirming that their daily activities were productive and their lifestyles less stressful when they incorporated the Christ-like self-identity tools they learned. For example, the group participants commented that their ongoing redefining on their lifestyle from childhood through adulthood helped them to understand reactions and responses toward self and others. The participants confirmed that the session reassured their belief and trust that their self-identity is found within the Scripture and confession of God's Word. Their comments in response to the qualitative questions mentioned that the woman of valor within Proverbs 31 illustrated the type of character needed, and assisted them with their daily interactions with family members, co-workers, and strangers. The participants agreed that The Diva's proclamation prepared them for their daily activities, and that the song "I Know Who I Am" reminded them of their identity in Christ and provided strength to endure life challenges.

As I reflect back, I believed the workshop permitted each woman to have an inward and outward understanding of her self-value in Christ. The effective result from this self-identity through redefining one's identity in Christ stirred me continue to mimic Christ and to continue to offer workshops that encourage women to overcome their understanding of their identity through God's Divine Wellness Plan.

Application

The feedback received from the six-week session revealed the benefit of the workshop for participants within their personal, professional and social lifestyles. I felt truly grateful and honored to be able to use my holistic expertise given to me through God's grace to assist others on their wellness journey.

To build upon this project, I would be interested in incorporating two additional extension sessions, one advanced project, and a buddy system. A project B, an extension from the first one, could either be an additional time every six weeks or a monthly interactive workshop, expanding on the material provided within the first series of workshops. For example, during the Healthy Heart Soul-Searching session, more time could have been given to each subtitle. The soul-searching session could have been divided into mini interactive workshop. This would have allowed the participants to share their emotional concerns in relation to their daily challenges. The soul-searching workshop was very intense, and the women expressed how they were delivered from feelings of shame and guilt.

A workshop could also be designed to focus on Lament Prayer. This class would divide the time between the illustrations of the various emotions found within the prayers in Psalms, allowing them to write out their prayers during the session rather than only doing so as a homework assignment. It would have allowed time for discussion of the participants' Lament Prayers which would have been beneficial to the group.

Third, I am also interested in designing a project two for returning participants. This would assist the women in their wellness walk as women of character who are growing in God's grace. These six to eight-week sessions would enhance their spiritual understanding by more in-depth study in God's word, particularly on Proverbs 31:10-31. Since their faith walk is ongoing, this would encourage and aid them in areas that still challenge them.

I would structure this type of group in a way similar to a book club, within an interactive workshop environment. The sessions would incorporate discussion of the assigned chapters, yet the class format would be creatively designed to educate, encourage personal sharing, and provide a trusting environment. The workshops would be strategically designed to include role plays, games, meditations, videos, power point presentations, and guest speakers. I would potentially integrate the following books in this type of program:

Demoss, Nancy Leigh. 2001. *Lies Women Believe and the Truth That Sets Them Free*. Chicago, IL: Moody Publishers.

George, Elizabeth.1997. *Women After God's Own Heart*. Eugene, OR: Harvest House Publishers.

McCloud, Melody T. M.D. 2010. *Living Well… Despite Catchin' Hell: The Black Woman's Guide to Health, Sex & Happiness*. Roswell, GA: New Life Publishing.

Finally, I would add a buddy system within the workshop sessions. In my observation of the interaction among the participants during and after class sessions, I noticed how they remained in groups during break times and while socializing after class in the parking lot. A buddy system would pair the women to be motivator, accountability person, and prayer partner to each other throughout the six weeks of sessions. This will give them a chance to make new acquaintance and fellowship.

In regards to my on-going ministry, I am planning to host a Diva's mother and daughter summer camp and have incorporated break-out discussion sessions in my planning. These sessions will give the participants more time to communicate the various areas of concerns they are having on the discussion topic as I engage in active listening. To assist the women in relating to their daughters, which was a relationship concern, there will be fun activities for mother and daughter. This energetic, fun, and educational summer camp will incorporate an understanding of the traditional upbringing of African American women, the recognition of prominent African American women, and the need for self-acceptance in society.

I understand that to help women seek, find and accept their Christ-like identity, I must continue to seek God to improve my overall health and wellbeing while continuing to seek further education in the area of wellness. I have also learned that in order to promote total wellness and to inspire women of all ages to love, respect and appreciate their self-identity in Christ, I must submit to the Holy Spirit's guidance in the areas of discerning collective and individual holistic needs.

Further Study

Three avenues of further study would be beneficial to pursue. When studying mental health rates among African Americans, I became aware of the high percentage of African American women who were diagnosed with mental illnesses. More extensive research can be done on the historical adverse affects on the holistic lifestyles of African American women in the following areas: psychological distress in relation to income status, emotional stress in relation to unemployment, mental illnesses, especially in the form of bipolar disorder and clinical depression, and physical difficulties because of the lack of affordable healthcare.

A research project could also be implemented to identify the beliefs and attitudes of African American women toward behaviors necessary for good mental health. Primary care providers, medications, social services, pastoral services, and informal support and avoidance should be addressed in the research project.

Finally, it would be important to compare the historical records that give insight into those African American women who have been able to achieve transformation within their lifestyle practices. Incorporating personal interviews of women today, who have served in various roles, such as civil rights activists, educational advocates, entertainers, health care professionals, and housewives, could provide valuable information and guidance to the design of support systems for those who continue to struggle. This would give insight into the perspective of African American women and their experiences within their various lifestyle challenges.

Personal Goals

Our vision is to build communities by improving the lifestyles of women, one women at a time. Our mission is to promote total wellness and to inspire women of all ages through fashion as they accept and become confident in their unique, wonderful, spiritual, and physical image.

The above is the mission statement of the project; Diva's Lifestyle Identity Journey, and is my goal to achieve wellness in my own lifestyle. My daily activities and choices were no longer mine, and, therefore, public. They were on display and subject to the critique of Scripture. This reminded me that since I chose to help other African American women concerning how to live within God's Divine Wellness plan, my personal lifestyle choices were no longer my own. I took on the responsibility to motivate the African American women to "follow my example as I follow the example of Christ" (1 Corinthians 11:1). This meant I had to make sure my personal goals would be subject to my nightly spiritual and physical check-ups in light of God's wellness plan for me.

At this point in this reflection, I will address my four personal goals for this project: My first goal was to make a greater impact in my spiritual life through intensive integration of spiritual and physical disciplines; second, to develop a closer relationship with God through intimate relationship with Him; third, to accept people's choices when I do not agree with them; and fourth, to make sure I accept others' viewpoint.

Personal Goal Number One

Spiritual Life Impact: Intensive Integration Spiritual and Physical Discipline

My first personal goal was to make a greater spiritual life impact through intensive integration through spiritual and physical discipline. This was to make sure I practiced what I preached. Avoiding mediocrity within my daily activities was possible when I kept my eyes on Jesus. The woman of character in Proverbs 31: 15 rose early and provided for her household, and her example became a part of my morning ritual. In the morning while I am preparing my husband's meals for work, I had started seeking the Holy Spirit's guidance on meal preparation and communication skill for early morning interaction with family members.

Also, I have integrated the following spiritual and physical discipline: 1. During my morning health and fitness routine, I have incorporated Scripture proclamation of whom I am in Christ while walking on the treadmill; 2. I am seeking God's guidance on how to serve others with compassion, kindness, humility, and patients (Col. 3:12); 3. I am taking prayer breaks throughout the day for wisdom on word choices, decisions, forgiveness, and bearing with others (Col. 3: 13-14). I can see how I have made progress. I am enjoying the restoration of spiritual and physical balance. In order to maintain this balance, I intentionally seek God before any decisions, whether they are emotional, physical, financial, or spiritual discipline, while engaging in a more intimate relationship with God.

Personal Goal Number Two
Intimate Relationship with God

My second goal was to become more intimate with God. My personal Diva's Lifestyle Identity experience has helped my intimate relationship with God as my prayer life increased. I continuously sought God to make sure my lifestyle revolved around His characteristics, yet I noticed I was not spending enough time with God giving Him adoration. Now, during my fitness routine, I play worship music and praise Him. Throughout my day, I set aside time to worship Him by verbally

90

proclaiming various praise and worship Scriptures. I have added evening Bible study time to learn more about His goodness. My time spent with God was not giving God glory.

My additional time spent in intimacy with God has become visual as follows: 1. Helped in my interactions with others (Col. 3:17), 2. Noticeable in my spoken words of boldness, love in faith towards others (Prov. 31: 8-9; 26); 3. Revealed within my praise and worship lifestyle (Prov. 31:10-31). Since I walked in the visually true beauty found within Christ, I must be in acceptance of others' choices (Prov. 31:25; Col. 3: 12 and 17).

Personal Goal Number Three
Acceptance of Other's Choices

My third goal was to become more accepting of others' choices. This area has produced great growth in controlling my speech. I noticed that when the participants' choices went against the wellness teaching, I was able to listen carefully and to call on Jesus to see if I needed to respond in love by offering constructive feedback. I was able to ask myself whether they needed more clarification about the wellness teaching due to their misunderstanding or did I need to be more receptive of their opinions about the information.

As I have been seeking God in prayer for the solution to the acceptance of other's choices, He reminded me that His love is not judgmental and that He has given me the opportunity to share His wellness plan versus condemning their current lifestyle. What has helped me to accept other's choice is the Holy Spirit's voice that reminds me that His grace is sufficient for me. I have not always made the choices that glorified God. I am still growing in God's grace on this assignment.

Personal Goal Number Four
Acceptance of Other's Viewpoint

My final goal was to become more accepting of others' viewpoints. This is an ongoing practice for me. This project has helped me to grow within my spiritual discipline of practicing God's love through relationships. I am relying on my walk in faith and not on the self-perception based upon my own opinion. One example was my response to the suggestion of others in relation to the marketing strategies used to solicit participants from various community outreach centers. At first, I was apprehensive of some of the suggestions that I thought might be time-consuming. Through prayer, God reminded me that my ways are not the only ways to reach the target market. Now, I can say that I am more accepting of the suggestions of others without placing them within my self-made categories. I have incorporated a daily prayer where I proclaim that I will not take things personally and be open to God's constructive criticism through others.

While not part of my written goals for this project, it has been my hope that the Diva's Lifestyle Identity Journey could continue beyond this six-week project. Hopefully with funding from a continuous grant, this project will transition into ongoing six-week workshops throughout Ward 2, Cleveland Ohio.

Concluding Thoughts

The impact workshop's mission improved the lifestyle of women, one woman at a time. Each woman commented on how Diva's Total Wellness Plan inspired them through the fashion show, stress meditation, daily devotional, ongoing prayer, and group support. The women's core value of self-identity was rooted upon their faith values and knowledge of who they are. The challenges of life built their character, and improved their unique and wonderful image in Christ, both spiritually and physically. The women were excited at the ability to accept ownership over their thought processes, which was a major component of discovering who they are.

The Bible-based approach to a holistic lifestyle successfully unified the participants in spirit, soul, and body as they interacted with the various components of wellness: nutrition intake, physical movements, emotional stability, stress release, financial management, and social interaction. The holistic health approach throughout the impact workshop helped the African American women to comprehend that their well-being is rooted in maintaining a balance between mind and body versus one in lordship over the other.

This is why I believe a better term for the approach would be Wholistic rather than Holistic. God's wellness plan permits His people to worship and serve Him with a Wholistic fitness of body, mind and soul. Society's Holistic lifestyle incorporates the concept of holism in relation to wholeness; yet, the stronger wellness components rule in relation to one's life circumstances.

The workshops aided the African American women in proclaiming that they can be satisfied with the physical image of their body because their bodies coincide with their biological and genetic makeup. The Body Image session revealed their healthy self-image in Christ. After the Mouth Trap session, they stated that they were more aware that death and life is contained within the power of their tongues. The dress style session gave them the visual image on who they appeared to be in Christ. Finally, the interactive workshop reminded the women to continue to evolve. African American women were encouraged to continue on their wellness journey through ongoing educational courses on how to maintain a lifestyle that will shine through in their dress attire, which portrayed a part of their holistic image.

A woman's fashion statement portrays a part of her holistic image. Her style builds and represents her self-confidence and provides the world with a snapshot of her unique, wonderful, spiritual and physical image (Weems, 2016, 98).

As I continue in my personal wellness journey, the theme song, "I Know Who I Am" encourages and motivates me to appreciate and respect who I am in Christ. This has been an energizing, exciting, and challenging journey. My self-identity in Christ has provided me with internal motivation and encouraged me to seek an ongoing Bible-based wellness lifestyle. This was the driving force behind my compassion and desire to educate others on how to maintain a healthy fashionable lifestyle according to God's divine wellness plan, and remains my passion at the end of this phase of my journey.

APPENDIX
A DIVA'S Lifestyle Identity JOURNEY
IMPROVING THE LIFESTYLE OF A WOMAN

ONE WOMAN AT A TIME

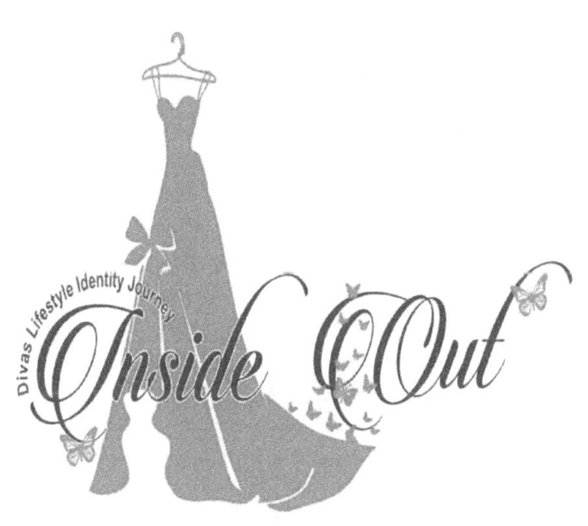

RECOMMEND BY ESTHER INTERNATIONAL INC.

REVEREND FREDINA USHER-WEEMS, M Div, Ba/Ed

<u>INSIDE OUT/DIVA'S LIFESTYLE IDENTITY</u>
<u>WEEK 1: ORIENTATION/PROJECT OVERVIEW</u>

Welcome!
Welcome to our creatively and uniquely designed 6 weeks Inside/Out/Diva's Lifestyle Identity Journey program. We are here to help you on your wholistic journey. We pray and believe that the motivation and encouragement you received through our wellness tools will energize and transition you from your current crisis or situation into a healthy lifestyle which will reveal the awakening of your true self in the following healthy characteristics of a Diva:
Week 1: Orientation/Stress Release
 Week 2: Identity Crisis: Who am I?
 Week 3: Healthy Heart/Soul
 Week 4: Fitness/Body Image
 Week 5: Mouth Trap: Word Choices
 Week 6: Dress for Success/Diva's Wrap up

Introduction
We would like to introduce you to your support persons, motivators, friend, and facilitators
1. Shuywanna Ford
2. Reverend Fredina Weems, known as Fredi.

Additional Information
You can give us as much information as you fill comfortable. The more you give us the more we will be able to assist you.
This information will be kept confidential and only your truly, the facilitator will view the files.
This will help us understand your health condition, nutrition like dislikes, allergy, fitness history, spiritual preference, hobbies, and any other personal information you think we should know.

GROUP SESSION DECORUM:

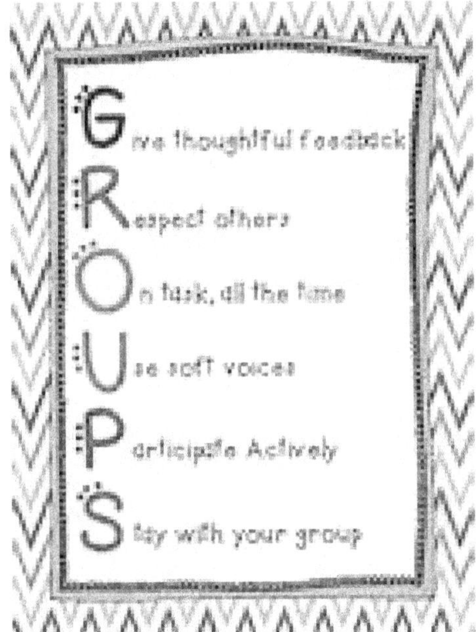

Diva's Decorum

Also, Sideline Rules
- Be prompt
- Do NOT repeat what is shared in the group
- Hug when necessary
- Back off when others are pushed too far
- Don't make excuses Own Up
Restroom

Stress Release Exercise
Tai Chi or 3 R's

Diva's Proclamation
Look into your personalized mirror repeat after your facilitator:
I am strong! I have been and will continue to be.
I am happy! I do not depend on others to make me happy. I am in a daily pursuit of fulfilling my purpose and that makes me happy.
I am successful! I have achieved by leaps and bounds in my life and there are many more to come in the future!
I am amazing! I am good enough, beautiful and a wonderful person.
Most of all, **I LOVE ME!**

Stress

Let take self-evaluation; stress level.

Is how your body response to life challenges; dangerous, threatening, surprise, joyous, grief, etc. We all handle stress differently.

Historical

African American ways of coping with adversity has been passed down through our parents since slavery. Stoicism and silent suffering were the learned behavior our ancestors used to overcome threats to their survival.

Today we use the same behavior to cope with various stressful situations

1. Eliminate Stress
2. Sleep
3. Smoking
4. Review your list of stressors in perspective

SELF-EVALUATION: YOUR STRESS LEVEL

Purpose

To see if you need healthier ways to relieve stress.

Stress Scale

Respond to each statement using the following scale:

5 = strongly agree 4 = agree   3 = neutral 2 = disagree 1 = strongly disagree

Stress Questions

1.   I find it hard to get more than three or four hours of sleep a night.
2.   I've tried to quit smoking, but every time I face situation I light up.
3.   I get upset, I tend to eat more.
4.   I feel challenged (work, home, etc.) I panic.
5. I have a great deal of stress in my life, but I just hold it in because I don't want to burden anyone with my troubles.

How are you dealing with stress? A score of 5 indicates that you're doing great job handling stress. If your score is closer to 25, just need to prayerfully seek wisdom on how to handle your stress level.

Journal Entries

Your journal entries which are required for each session are to help you to understand what's going on inside you. It's extremely important for each one of you to experience your own unique emotional journey. You should expect to expand your mind in the following areas: what is going on in your mind, notating your strong and weak areas, releasing your feelings, recording your progress, brain storming, and making decisions. We will be reviewing your journal and offering some suggestions to assist you on your Diva's Lifestyle Journey.

Journal entries are required for each session.
Why?
To help you understand what is going on inside you.
Journaling will help to expand your mind in the following areas:
1. Releasing your feelings
2. What is going on in your mind
3. Notating your strong and weak areas
4. Recording your progress
5. Brain storming
6. Making decisions

You will be learning more about that during our next sessions.

Homework Assignment
1. Journal
   a. Go home and write a journal entry.
   b. Freely express your thoughts about your day, impact made, stress
   c. Where you thought, you could have done better
   d. Feeling creative write, a poem or short story to share with the class.
2. Make your faith declaration daily
3. Read your Daily Bread each day
4. Pick out jewelry or clothing favorite to wear next week and be prepared to discuss in 2-3 minutes why you love the jewelry or clothing
   a. Ex. Does this item reflect your personality for this day
   b. Ex. Makes you feel close to a loved one

Summary
Ms. Divas, these sessions will assist and prepare you for a positive productive future regardless of your life challenges if you are willing to do the footwork (smile Diva) We are looking forward to assisting you on your wholistic journey (spirit, soul, and body)

Let's end by proclaiming
I know who I am.

REFERENCES

Adams, Jay E. 1986. *The Biblical View of Self-Esteem Self-Love Self-Image*.
Eugene, OR: Harvest House Publisher.

Afrika, Llaila O. 2004. *African Holistic Health*. 7th ed. Brooklyn, NY: A&B Publishers
Group.

Anekwe, Obiora N. Ed. 2015. Artist's Statement: Tuskegee Men. *Academic
Medicine*. Volume 90(5), (May 2015): 621. (Accessed March 29, 2017).

Ansberry, C. B. 2010. What Does Jerusalem Have to Do with Athens?" The Moral
Vision of the Book of Proverbs and Aristotle's Nicomachean Ethics. *Hebrew
Studies* 51, 157-173.

Barclay, William. 1961. *The All-Sufficient Christ: Studies in Paul's Letter to The
Colossians*. Philadelphia, PA: Westminster Press.

Beetham, Christopher A. 2010. *Echoes of Scripture in the Letter of Paul to the
Colossians*. Atlanta, GA: Society of Biblical Literature.

Benner, David, G. 2001. *Spirituality and the Awakening Self: The Sacred Journey of
Transformation*. Grand Rapids, MI: Brazos.

Betts, Kate. 2011. *Everyday ICON: Michelle Obama and the Power of Style*. New
York, NY: Clarkson Potter Publisher.

Bills, E.R. 2014. *The 1910 Slocum Massacre: An Act of Genocide in East Texas*.
Charleston, SC: The History Press.

Biscoglio, Frances Minetti. 1993. *The Wives of The Canterbury: Tales and Tradition
of The Valiant Woman of Proverbs 31:10-31*. San Francisco, CA: Mellen
Research University Press.

Biwul, Joel Kamsen Tihitshak. 2013. Reading the Virtuous Woman of Proverbs
31:10-31 as a Reflection of the Attributes of the Traditional Miship Woman of
Nigeria 1. JosEcwa Theological Seminary. Old testam. essays vol.26 n.2
Pretoria Jan. 2013 275-297.
http://www.scielo.org.za/scielo.php?script=sci_arttext&pid=S1010-
99192013000200005.

Bond, Beverly. 2006. "Break Through Women: Black Girls Rock."
http://www.blackgirlsrockinc.com/home/#.WXIk8WLyvIW. (accessed July 21,
2017).

Boyd, Gregory, A. 2010. *Present Perfect: Finding God in the Now*. Grand Rapids,
MI: Zondervan.

Branch Gallaher, R. 2012. Proverbs 31:10-31: A Passage Containing Wisdom
Principles for a Successful Marriage. *Koers-Bulletin for Christian Scholarship*
77(2), Art #49. 9 pages. http://dx.doi.org/104102/koers.v77/2.49. (Accessed
July 16, 2017).

Bruce. F.F. 1977. *Paul: Apostle of the Heart Set Free*. Grand Rapids, MI: William B.
Eerdmans Publishing Company.

Bultmann, Rudolf. 1951.*Theology of the New Testament*. 2 vols. New York: Charles
Scribner's Sons.

Byrd, Ayana and Akiba Solomon. 2005. *Naked: Black Women Bare All About Their
Skin, Hair, Hips, Lips, and Other Parts*. New York, NY: Penguin Group
Publisher.

Byrd, Michael W. and Linda A. Clayton. 2000. *An American Health Dilemma: A
Medical History of African Americans and The Problems of Race Beginnings
to 1900*. New York, NY: Routledge Publications.

________. 2011. Race, Medicine, and Health Care in the United States: A Historical
Survey. *Journal of National Medical Association*. Vol. 94 No. 3 (SUPPL)115-
345.

Cahill, Lisa Sowle. 1992. *Women and Sexuality*. Mahwah, NJ: Paulist Press.

Carmody, John. 1983. *Holistic Spirituality*. Ramsey, NJ: Paulist Press.

Carson, D.A. 1991. *The Gospel According to John*. The Pillar New Testament
Commentary, ed. Grand Rapids, MI: William B. Eerdmans Publishing
Company.

Carter, Norvella, Ph.D. and Matthew Parker. 1996. *Women to Women: Perspectives of Fifteen African-American Christian Women*. Grand Rapids, MI: Zondervan Publishing House.

Cash, Thomas F. and Thomas Pruzinsky. 2002. *Body Image: A Handbook of Theory, Research, and Clinical Practice*. New York, NY: The Guilford Press.

Chan, Simon. 1998. *Spiritual Theology: A Systematic Study of the Christian Life.* Downer Grove, IL: InterVarsity Press.

Chase, Deborah. 1996. *Fruit Acids for Fabulous Skin*. New York, NY: St. Martin's Paperbacks.

Childs, Brevard S. 1985. *Old Testament Theology in a Canonical Context.* Philadelphia, PA: Fortress Press.

Coleman, Monica A. 2008. *Making a Way Out of No Way: A Womanist Theology.* Minneapolis, MN: Fortress Press.

__________. 2016. *Bipolar Faith: A Black Woman's Journey with Depression and Faith*. Minneapolis, MN: Fortress Press.

Collins, Catherine Fisher. 2013. *African American Women's Life Issues Today: Vital Health and Social Matters*. Santa Barbara, CA: Praeger An Imprint of ABC-CLIO, LLC.

Committee on Diet and Health; Food and Nutrition Board. 1989. *Diet and Health: Implications for Reducing Chronic Disease Risk.* Washington, D.C.: National Academy Press. 563-592.

Cornish, Grace, Dr. 2002. *10 Good Choices That Empower Black Women's Lives.* New York, NY; Random House.

Cotton, Richard, T. and Robert, L. Goldstein. 1993. *Aerobics Instructor Manual: The Resource for Fitness Professionals*. San Diego, CA: American Council on Exercise Publication.

Craig, U-Shaka. 2013. *Shifting Your Paradigm For Optimum Health and Longevity: A Model of Health and Healing for African Americans*. Albermarle, NC: Gye Nyame Publishing House

Crowther, Nigel B. 2010. *Sports in Ancient Times*. Norman, OK: University of Oklahoma Press.

Davis, Ellen F. 2000. *Proverbs, Ecclesiastes, and the Song of Songs*. Louisville, KY: John Knox Press.

DeFranza, Megan. 2011. The Proverbs 31: "Woman of Strength: An Argument for a Primary Sense Translation. *The Priscilla Papers*. 25 (2) Winter. 17-20.

Derosis, Helen. M.D. 1998. *Women and Anxiety: A Step-by-Step Program for Managing Anxiety and Depression*. 2nd ed. New York, NY: Hatherleigh Press.

Downs, Jim. 2012. *Sick from Freedom: African-American Illnesses and Suffering During Civil War and Reconstruction*. New York, NY: Oxford University Press.

Dube, Musa, W. 2001. *Other Ways of Reading: African Women and the Bible*. Atlanta, GA: WCC Publication.

Dula, Anette and Sara Goering. 1994. *It Just Ain't Fair: The Ethics of Health Care for African Americans*. Westport, CT: Praeger Publication.

Ehlke, Roland. 1992. *Proverbs*. The People Bible Commentary. St. Louis MO: Concordia Publishing House.

Eising, Hermann. 1980. *Theological Dictionary of the Old Testament*, vol. !V. ed. G. Johannes Botterweck and Helmer Ringgren, trans. David E. Green. Grand Rapids, MI: Eerdmans.

Ellison, Marvin M. and Kelly Brown Douglas. 2010. *Sexuality and the Sacred: Source for Theological Reflection*. 2nd ed. Louisville, KY: Westminster John Knox Press.

Elwell, Walter A. 2001. *Evangelical Dictionary of Theology*. 2nd ed. Grand Rapids, MI: Baker Academic Publication.

Erickson, Mildred J. 1998 *Christian Theology*. 2nd ed. Grand Rapids, MI: Baker Academic Publication.

Esselstyn. Caldwell B. Jr. 2008. *Prevent and Reverse Heart Disease: The Revolutionary, Scientifically Proven, Nutrition-Based Cure.* New York, NY: Penguin Group Publication.

Exum, J. Cheryl. 1994. You Shall Let Every Daughter Live: A Study of Exodus 1:8-2:10. In *A Feminist Companion to Exodus to Deuteronomy.* Athayla Brenner, ed. 37-61. Sheffield, England: Sheffield University Press.

Feldstein, Ruth. 2013. *How It Feels to Be Free; Black Women Entertainers and the Civil Rights Movement.* New York, NY: Oxford University Press.

Ferrell, Pamela. 1996. *Let's Talk Hair.* Washington, DC: Conrow Publisher.

Fitzpatrick, Carol, L. 2014. *The Best of Daily Wisdom for Women.* Uhrichsville, OH: Barbour Publishing, Inc.,

Forbes, Ella. 1998. *African American Women During the Civil War.* New York, NY: Garland Publishing, Inc.,

Fornay, Alfred. 2002. *The African American Woman's Guide to Successful Makeup and Skincare.* New York, NY: John Wiley & Sons, Inc.

Foster, Richard J. 2008. *Life with God: Reading the Bible for Spiritual Transformation.* New York, NY: HarperCollins Publishers.

__________.2008. *The Attentive Life: Discerning God's Presence in All Things.* Downer Grove, IL: InterVarsity Press.

Fox, Michael V. 2009. *Proverbs 10-31: A New Translation with Introduction and Commentary.* Binghamton, NY: Vail-Ballou Press.

George, Elizabeth. 2014. *Beautiful In God's Eyes: For Young Women Looking Good from the Inside Out.* Eugene, OR: Harvest Brown Publishers.

Green. Joel B. 2008. *Body, Soul, And Human Life: The Nature of Humanity in the Bible.* Grand Rapids, MI: Baker Publishing Group.

Golubic, Mladen. Dr. 2016. Interview by Reverend Fredina J. Weems. OH. December 5.

Gourdine, Michelle A. 2011. *Reclaiming Our Health: A Guide to African American Wellness*. New Haven: Yale University Press.

Gundry, Patricia. 1981. *The Complete Woman: Being A Whole Person*. Garden City, NY: Doubleday Publication.

Haggard, Dixie Ray. 2010. *African Americans in the Nineteenth Century: People and Perspectives*. Denver, CO: ABC-CLIO, LCC.

Hartley, John E. 2016. *Proverbs: A Commentary in the Wesleyan Tradition*. Kansas City, MO: Beacon Hill Press.

Hill, Shirley, A. 2016. *Inequality and African-American Health: How Racial Disparities Create Sickness*. Chicago, IL: Policy Press.

Hogue, Carol, J.R., Martha A. Hargraves, and Karen Scott Collins. 2000. *Minority Health in America: Findings and Policy Implications from Commonwealth Fund Minority Health Survey*. Baltimore, MD: The John Hopkins University Press.

Hooks, Bell. 2015. *Sisters of the Yam: Black Women and Self-Recovery*. New York, NY: Routledge Publisher.

Hollies, Linda H. 2003. *Bodacious Womanist Wisdom*. Cleveland OH: Pilgrims Press.

Hoytt, Eleanor Hinton and Hilary Beard. 2012. *Health First! The Black Woman's Wellness Guide*. New York, NY: Hay House, Inc.

Hull, Gloria T., Patricia Bell Scott, and Barbara Smith. 1982. *All the Women are White, All the Blacks are Men: But Some of Us are Brave, Black Women Studies*. New York, NY: The Feminist Press at the City University of New York.

Jack, Leonard, Jr. 2010. *Diabetes in Black America: Public Health and Clinical Solutions to a National Crisis*. Roscoe, IL: Hilton Publishing Company.

Johnson, Beverly. 1994. *True Beauty: Secrets of Radiant Beauty for Women of Every Age and Color*. US: Warner Books Publication.

Johnson, Karen A., Abul Pitre, and Kenneth L. Johnson. 2014. *African American Women Educators: A Critical Examination of Their Pedagogies Educational Ideals and Activism from Nineteenth to the Mid-Twentieth Century.* Lanham, MD: Rowman & Littlefield Education, A Division of Rowman & Littlefield.

Johnson, Naomi. 2013. "My Black is Beautiful." http://www.powerpoetry.org/poems/my-black-beautiful-3-woman. (accessed June 30, 2017)

Johnson, Yvonne. 1998. *The Voices of African American Women: The Use of Narrative and Authorial Voice in the Works of Harriet Jacobs, Zora Neale Hurston, and Alice Walker.* New York, NY: Peter Lang Publishing.

Kanyoro. Musimbi R.A. 2002. *Introducing Feminist Cultural Hermeneutics: An African Perspective.* Cleveland, OH: The Pilgrim Press.

Karen Kruse. 2011. *Deluxe Jim Crow: Civil Rights and American Policy*, 1935-1954. Athens, GA: The University of Georgia Press.

Katzman, David M. 1973. *Before the Ghetto: Black Detroit in the Nineteenth Century.* Chicago, IL: University of Illinois Press.

Kebaneilwe, Mmapula Diana. 2012. *This Courageous Woman: A Socio-rhetorical Womanist Reading of Proverbs 31:10-31.* Murdoch University. http://researchrepository.murdoch.edu.au/id/eprint/16159/2/02Whole.pdf.

Koptak, Paul E. 2003. *Proverbs:* The NIV Application Commentary. Grand Rapids, MI: Zondervan.

Knowles, Beyoncé. 2016. "Beyoncé All-Night Lemonade" (video) November 30, 2016 https://www.youtube.com/watch?v=gM89Q5Eng_M&list=PLxKHVMqMZqUSP F11Ghs0KqDfOGhB9Vw5E. (accessed July 19, 2016).

Ladd, George Eldon. 1974. *A Theology of the New Testament.* Grand Rapids, MI: Eerdmans Publication.

Library of Congress.2013. *An Illustrated Guide. African-American History and Culture.* http:/www.loc.gov/rr/mss/guide/afrcan.html. (accessed June 4, 2017).

Lockley, Tim. 2013. Black Mortality in Antebellum Savannah. *Society History of Medicine*. Vol. 26, No. 4. 633-652.

Long, Gretchen. 2012. *Doctoring Freedom: The Politics of African American Medical Care in Slavery and Emancipation*. Chapel Hill, NC: The University of North Carolina Press.

Longman, Tremper, ed. 2006. *Baker Commentary on the Old Testament: Wisdom and Psalms.* Grand Rapids, MI: Baker Books.

Lowe, Tony B. 2006. Nineteenth Century Review of Mental Health Care for African Americans: A Legacy of Service and Policy Barriers. *The Journal of Sociology & Social Welfare* Volume 33, Article 5, 4(December): 29-50. http://scholarworks.wmich.edu/cgi/viewcontent.cgi?article=3202&context=jssw.

Lynch, Annette. 1999. *Dress, Gender and Cultural Change: Asian American and African American Rites of Passage*. New York, NY: Berg Publication.

Magdalen, Margaret. 1990. *A Spiritual Check-Up: Avoiding Mediocrity in the Christian Life*. Great Britain. Highland Books.

Martin, Ralph A.1973. *Colossians: The Church's Lord and the Christian's Liberty*. Grand Rapids, MI: Zondervan Publishing House.

McCloud, Melody T. 2010. *Living Well...Despite Catchin' Hell: The Black Woman's Guide to Health, Sex & Happiness*. Roswell, GA: New Life Publishing.

McCloud, Melody T. and Angele Ebron. 2003. *Blessed Health: The African American Woman's Guide to Physical and Spiritual Well-Being*. New York, NY: Simon & Schuster Publication.

McConville, Gordon J. 2016. *Being Human in God's World: An Old Testament Theology of Humanity*. Grand Rapids, MI: Baker Academic, a Division of Baker Publishing Group.

McCurary, Crystal and Nathan Hale Williams. 2012. *Inspiration: Profiles of Black Women Changing Our World*. New York, NY: Stewart, Tabori & Chang Publication.

McGee, Robyn. 2005. *Hungry for More: Keeping-It-Real Guide for Black Women on Weight and Body Image*. Emeryville, CA: Seal Press Publication.

McQuirter, Tracye Lynn. 2010. *By Any Greens Necessary: A Revolutionary Guide for Black Women Who Want to Eat Great, Get Healthy, Lose Weight, and Look Phat*. Chicago IL: Lawrence Hill Books.

McMillen, S.I. and David E. Stern, 2000. *None of These Diseases: The Bible's Health Secrets for the 21st Century*. 3rd ed. Grand Rapids, MI: Fleming H. Revell.

Mitchem, Stephanie Y. 2002. *Introducing Womanist Theology*. Maryknoll, NY: Orbis Books Publication.

__________. 2004. *African American Women: Tapping Power and Spiritual Wellness*. Cleveland OH: The Pilgrim Press.

__________. 2007. *African American Folk Healing*. New York, NY: New York University Press.

Moltmann, Jürgen.1985. *God in Creation: A New Theology of Creation and the Spirit of God*. San Francisco: Harper and Row Publication.

__________.1993. *Theology of Hope: On the Ground and Implication of Christian Eschatology*. Minneapolis, MN: Fortress Press.

Moltmann, Jürgen and Elisabeth Moltmann-Wendel. 1990. *The Way of Jesus Christ*. London: SCM Press.

__________. 1991. *GOD – His and Hers*. New York, NY: Crossroad Publisher.

__________. 2003. *Passion for God: Theology in Two Voices*. Louisville, KY: Westminster John Knox Press.

Moreland, J.P. & Scott B. Rae. *Body and Soul: Human Nature & the Crisis in Ethics*. 2000. Downer Groves, IL: InterVarsity Press.

Morgante, James. Toward A Theology of Wellness; Health, in the Judeo-Christian Tradition, Is Understood Holistically and Connected to the State of One's Relationship to God. *Health Progress*, (Nov/Dec 2002); ProQuest Central, 19-21. Accessed October 17, 2014. http://search.proquest.com.ezproxy.liberty.edu:2048/docview/274402953?pq-origsite=summon.

Moss, Cheryl Talley. 1999. *Healthy Hair Care Tips for Today's Black Woman*. Mesquite, TX: Talley Publishing.

Moule, C.F.D. 1957. *The Epistles of Paul the Apostle to the Colossians and to Philemon*. The Cambridge Greek Testament Commentary, Cambridge: Hodder and Stoughton.

Musgrave, Catherine F., Carol Easley Allen, and Gregory J. Allen. 2002. Spirituality and Health for Women of Color. *American Journal of Public Health*, April. 92(4) 557-560.

Neal-Barnett, Angela. 2003. *Soothe Your Nerves: The Black Woman's Guide to Understanding and Overcoming Anxiety, Pain, and Fear*. New York, NY: Simon & Schuster Publication.

Norton, Amy. 2011. Healthy Waist May Be a Bit Bigger for Black Women. *Reuters Health* January. http://www.reuters.com/article/us-healthy-waist-idUSTRE70O4H320110125. (accessed May 27, 2017).

Nygengele, Mpyana Fulgence. 2004. African Women's Theology, Gender Relations, and Family Systems Theory: Pastoral Theological Considerations and Guidelines for Care and Counseling. *America University Studies. Series VII. Theology and Religion*. New York, NY: Peter Lang Publication.

Ornish, Dean. 2007. *The Spectrum: A Scientifically Proven Program to Feel Better, Live Longer, Lose Weight, Gain Weight*. New York, NY: Ballantine Book.

Patterson, Sheron C. 2000. *New Faith: A Black Christian Woman's Guide to Reformation, Re-Creation, Rediscover, Renaissance, Resurrection, and Revival*. Minneapolis, MN: Fortress Press.

Peterson, Eugene, H. 2006. *Eat This Book: A Conversation in the Art of Spiritual Reading*. Grand Rapids, MI: William B. Eerdmans Publishing Company.

Richardson, Carolyn and Mary Hartley. 2011. Study Shows Black Women Can Be Healthy at Higher Weights. November. https://www.thoughtco.com/black-women-healthier-at-higher-weight-3533809 (accessed May 27, 2017).

Samuels, David. 2012. *Managed Health Care in the New Millennium: Innovative Financial Modeling for the 21 Century.* Boca Raton: CRC Press.

Sanders, Cheryl J. 1995. *Living the Intersection: Womanism and Afrocentrism In Theology.* Minneapolis, MN: Fortress Publishers.

Schwartz, Marie Jenkins. 2006. *Birthing A Slave: Motherhood and Medicine in the Antebellum South.* Cambridge MA: Harvard University Press.

Schwarz, Hans. 2013. *The Human Being: A Theological Anthropology.* Grand Rapids, MI: William B. Eerdmans Publishing Company.

Scott, A. Lear, Karen H. Humphries, Simi Kohl, and C. Laird Birmingham. 2007. "Use of BMI and Waist Circumference as Surrogates of Body Fat Differs by Ethnicity." *Obesity* Vol. 15 No. 11: 2817-2824. http://www.academia.edu/164314/Use_of_BMI_and_waist_circumference_as _surrogates_of_body_fat_differs_by_ethnicity. (accessed May 27, 2017).

Seamond, Stephen. 2003. *Wounds That Heal: Bringing Our Hurts to the Cross.* Downers Grove, IL: InterVarsity Press.

Shakir, Ameenah. African American Women Doctors In the Early 20th Century (Video). Lecture, Florida A&M University, 4/20/16, Accessed March 26, 2017. https://www.c-span.org/video/?408414-1/africanamerican-women-doctors-early-20th-century.

Sims, Naomi. 1982. *All About Success For The Black Woman.* Garden City, NY: Doubleday and Company, Inc.

Simundson, Daniel J. 1982. Health and Healing in the Bible. *Word & Word* Volume II Number 4 fall: 331-339http://proxy.ashland.edu:2328/ehost/detail/detail?vid=14&sid=423f10f-57f243a8-978a-4c85612dfd0%40sessionmgr4001&hid=4106&bdata=JnNpdGU9ZWhvc3Qtb G12ZQ%3d%3d#db=a6h&AN=ATLA00000795449(Accessed January 30, 2015).

Smith, George Edmond, M.D. 2001. *Weight Loss for African-American Women: An Eight-Week Guide to Better Health.* Roscoe, IL: Hilton Publishing Company.

Smith, Mitzi J. 2015. *I Found God in Me.* Eugene, OR: Wipf and Stock Publishers.

Swenson, Richard A. 2004. *Margin: Restoring Emotional, Physical, Financial, and Time Reserves to Overloaded Lives.* Colorado Springs, CO: NavPress.

Synge. F.C. 1958. *The Epistle of Paul The Apostle to The Philippians.* 2nd ed. Gateshead on Tyne, Great Britain: Northumberland Press Limited.

Tannenbaum, Rebecca J. 2012. *Health and Wellness in Colonial America.* Santa Barbara, CA: Greenwood Press.

Tarpley, Natasha. 1998. *Girl in the Mirror: Three Generations of Black Women in Motion.* Boston, MA. Beacon Press.

Taylor, Susan C. M.D. 2003. *Brown Skin: Dr. Susan Taylor's Prescription for Flawless Skin, Hair, and Nails.* New York, NY: HarperCollins Publishers Inc.

Thompson, Catherine, Rush. 2015. *Prevention Practice and Health Promotion: A Health Care Professional's Guide to Health, Fitness, and Wellness.* Thorofare, NJ: Slack Incorporated.

Thompson, Vincent Bakpetu.1987. *The Making of the African Diaspora in the American 1441-1900.* New York, NY: Longman Inc.

Thurman, Howard. 1996. *Jesus and the Disinherited.* Boston, MA: Beacon Press.

Tobert, Natalie, 2017. *Cultural Perspectives on Mental Wellbeing: Spiritual Interpretations of Symptoms in Medical Practices.* Philadelphia, PA: Jessica Kingsley Publishers

Villarosa, Linda. 1994. *Body and Soul: A National Black Women's Health Project Book.* Atlanta, GA: Harper Perennial Publication.

Vogelsang, TH. M. Leprosy in Norway, *Med Hist* (Jan 1965), 9(1), 29-35. Accessed October 22, 2014. http://www.ncbi.nlm.nih.gov/pmc/articles/PMC1033440/

Volo, James M. and Dorothy Denneen Volo. 2004. *The Antebellum Period: American Popular Culture Through History*. Westport, CT: Greenwood Press.

Von Speyr, Adrienne. 1998. *The Letter to the Colossians.* San Francisco, CA: Ignatius Press.

Wade, Felicia. 2014. BMI: Is the Scale Broken For Black Women? http://blackdoctor.org/451648/bmi-and-african-american-women__trashed/2/. (accessed May 30, 2017).

Washington, Harriet A. 2008. *Medical Apartheid: The Dark History of Medical Experiment on Black American From Colonial to the Present.* New York, NY: Anchor Press.

Wardle, Terry. 2001. *Healing Care Healing Prayer: Helping the Broken Find Wholeness in Christ.* Abilene, TX: Leafwood Publishers.

__________. 2016. "Identity Integrity and the Awakening of the True Self." Lecture, Ashland Theological Seminary, Ashland, OH, May 13, 2106.

Weems, Renita J. 1988. *Just A Sister Away: A Womanist Vision of Women's Relationships in the Bible*. San Diego, CA: LuraMedia Publication.

Weil, Andrew. 2012. *Life Is Your Best Medicine: A Woman's Guide to Health and Wholeness at Every Age*. Washington, DC.: National Geographic Society.

White, Augustus A. III, and David Chanoff. 2011. *Seeing Patients: Unconscious Bias in Health Care.* Cambridge, MA: Harvard University Press.

White, Evelyn, C. 1985. *Chain Chain Change: For Black Women Dealing with Physical and Emotional Abuse.* Seattle, WA: Evelyn White Publication.

Whitney, Donald S. 1991. *Spiritual Disciplines for the Christian Life.* Colorado Springs, CO: NavPress.

Whybray, R. N. 1995. *The Book of Proverbs: A Survey of Modern Study.* New York, NY: Kohn.

Willard, Dallas. 2012. *Renovation of the Heart*, 10th ed. Colorado Springs, CO: NavPress.

Wright. N.T. 2008. *Colossians and Philemon: Tyndale New Testament Commentaries*. Downer Grove, IL: InterVarsity Press.

ABOUT THE AUTHOR

Fredina Usher-Weems has a passion for the field of health and wellness. Her journey began at the young age of twelve when neighborhood friends and family members declared her the fitness instructor at the daycare center her parents owned in Cleveland, Ohio. When the kids came in, they started their morning off doing laps, jumping jacks, and push-ups.

She has a double major degree in Business Administration and in Health and Fitness. She also has a Master's degree in Art and Religion along with a Master of Divinity in Professionalism. She has a Wellness, Doctorate in Ministry from Ashland Theological Seminary. Her final ascent in education will be receiving a Master of Arts in Pastoral Counseling and Leadership.

While pursuing double majors in undergraduate studies, she taught aerobics classes, and gave health and fitness presentations at Cleveland area fitness centers. She also provided services to Girl Scout events, Cleveland Clinic's fitness facilities, Health Expression and the Cleveland Public School System. She holds several certifications including the American College of Sports Medicine, the Aerobic Fitness Association of America, and the Cooper Institute in Dallas, TX.

She currently carries the distinction of Distinguished Presenter in public speaking from Toastmasters International. She has been seen on local TV, written for Cleveland Clinic's Today's Daily Dose, The Health Hub Blog, and has contributed to the YouBeauty web site, The List (Channel Five) and other national publications. One of her greatest achievements however, was to find time to author her first wellness book called Fun Fitness: Living a Healthy Lifestyle and Having Fun.

Through her travels and thirty years of experience, she has developed a mantra: "Getting fit is about learning to love, respect, and appreciate you. Sometimes you fall, and that's ok!" Now, as a licensed Pastor/Minister, she is determined to maintain a healthy lifestyle, preach the Gospel through fitness, and educate and train others how to live a life of wellness based on biblical principles.

Dr. Usher-Weems can be reached at:

wonderfullymade 497@att.net and fredina@wonderfullymadeinc.com

website www.wonderfullymadeinc.com

www.ingramcontent.com/pod-product-compliance
Lightning Source LLC
Chambersburg PA
CBHW080026260726
48658CB00007B/2495